will yoga &
meditation
really change my life?

will yoga & meditation really change my life?

PERSONAL STORIES FROM 25 OF NORTH AMERICA'S LEADING TEACHERS

edited by Stephen Cope

A Kripalu BOOK

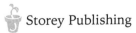 Storey Publishing

The mission of Storey Publishing is to serve our customers
by publishing practical information that encourages personal independence
in harmony with the environment.

Edited by Deborah Balmuth, Bhavani Lorraine Nelson,
    Atma Jo Ann Levitt, and Rachel Barenblat
Art direction by Cindy McFarland
Cover and text design by Susi Oberhelman
Cover photograph by Adam Mastoon
Text production by Jennifer Jepson Smith
Indexed by Danna Faulds
Photo credits are listed on page 321

Printed in the United States by R.R. Donnelley
10 9 8 7 6 5 4 3 2 1

Library of Congress Cataloging-in-Publication Data

Will yoga & meditation really change my life? : personal stories from
America's leading teachers / edited by Stephen Cope.
    p. cm.
  ISBN 1-58017-509-0 (alk. paper)
1. Meditation—Buddhism. 2. Spiritual biography—United States. 3.
Yoga. I. Title: Will yoga and meditation really change my life?. II.
Cope, Stephen.
BQ5612 .W56 2003
294.3'4432—dc22

2003014932

Contents

This volume is the first in a new series of Kripalu Books — a collaborative venture between Kripalu Center for Yoga & Health in Lenox, Massachusetts, and Storey Publishing in North Adams, Massachusetts. All royalties from this book will be donated to support the Diversity Scholarship Fund at Kripalu Center, helping to ensure that people from all walks of life can participate in contemplative practice.

Tales from the Path

How does contemplative practice — yoga and meditation — change us? Does it change our personalities, our biochemistry, our neurology, our deep mental structures? Or just, perhaps, our attitudes and beliefs? Does it change us at all, really, in any permanent sort of way?

These are questions that have been hovering in the background of my life, my work, and my imagination for at least the last fifteen years.

Throughout most of those years, I've been the Scholar-in-Residence and a senior instructor in yoga and meditation at Kripalu Center for Yoga & Health — one of the largest residential yoga centers in America. Perched high up in the Berkshire hills of Western Massachusetts, Kripalu has proved a remarkable vantage point from which to observe an astonishing explosion of interest in the Eastern contemplative traditions — particularly yoga and Buddhism. Each year Kripalu hosts over twenty-five thousand guests and hundreds of teachers who come to learn and teach techniques that they hope will allow them to live more fully.

Do these techniques work? Certainly, millions of people believe that they do. Their introduction into mainstream America has changed many of our ideas about spiritual life and spiritual practice — and is beginning to modify even our ideas about what is possible for human beings. Contemplative practice has now gained enough

influence in our culture to draw the interest of serious scientists —
psychologists, neurologists, and social scientists. I believe that in coming years we'll have some fascinating "hard" answers to my questions.

One thing is already certain, though: When the history of our
time is written, there will be important chapters about the transmission of the Eastern contemplative traditions onto Western
shores. What will these histories conclude? Will yoga and meditation
have changed our lives? Our culture? Do we have enough perspective yet to begin to make any meaningful responses to these
questions? I think we do. In fact, I think that in this historical
moment we have a very interesting perspective indeed.

I'm part of a significant slice of the "baby-boom generation"
of Americans who have now lived most of our adult lives deeply
influenced by contemplative practice. As I look around at my peers,
I realize that many of us are going gray, and contemplating our
retirement packages. Well, what do we have to say for ourselves?
How has thirty years of contemplative practice transformed us? How
has it transformed our lives, families, beliefs, bodies, interest in social
activism, sense of compassion, point of view about aging and death?

And on top of this, of course, comes another question: Is
thirty years a real perspective? I believe that it is. It seems to me that
this first generation of American contemplative practitioners holds
a fascinating piece of American spiritual and religious history.

Most of my fellow practitioners remember as I do the heady
days of the early 1970s, when yoga and meditation were exotic new
birds. In those years, I was a graduate student in theology at

Episcopal Divinity School in Cambridge, Massachusetts. It was a wild time to be studying theology: America was in the first flush of its romance with the contemplative traditions, and on any given Saturday evening you could meet your guru in Harvard Square. Chogyam Trungpa, Rinpoche, the great Tibetan teacher, had just decamped from England with his unique combination of crazy wisdom and elegant prose; Swami Muktananda, sporting his famous ostrich feather, was on his tour of America — astonishing students with his apparently supernormal powers; Swami Satchidananda had opened the Woodstock Festival and was already developing a large following of young American yogis; Joseph Goldstein, Jack Kornfield, and Sharon Salzberg were beginning to teach Vipassana meditation in a variety of venues in rural New England; and Suzuki Roshi was developing a whole generation of inspired Zen practitioners at the San Francisco Zen Center.

Thirty years have passed since those remarkable and colorful days. It's now quite clear that the transmission of the Eastern contemplative traditions onto American soil was not just a passing fad. Yoga has become the fastest growing practice in America — burgeoning from six million practitioners in 1994 to more than fifteen million today. Buddhism is one of the fastest growing religions on our continent. And the Western practice communities of these two traditions have become highly sophisticated — anchored as they are by a whole host of study centers, institutes, retreat centers, and centers for daily practice. These traditions are here to stay, and are now part of mainstream America.

Over the course of the past thirty years, a group of senior American teachers of both yoga and Buddhism has emerged. Many are teachers who came of age in the 1970s and have been serious practitioners ever since. Many have spent years on retreat and have engaged in serious practice with one or more authentic Eastern teachers. Many have joined ancient lineages, or founded their own communities. Most have spent a quarter of a century teaching and writing — taking seriously the challenge of transmitting these complex and sophisticated teachings to Western cultures.

> "What inspired you to become involved
> in contemplative practice,
> and what continues to be your deepest
> source of inspiration? What do you believe
> is possible for you 'in this very life'?"

During the past few years, I have found myself increasingly drawn to hearing the narratives of these long-term practitioners and teachers. And increasingly I have just one central question for them: "How has your practice changed your life?"

Fortunately, one aspect of my professional life has offered me a unique opportunity to ask that question of a great cross section of American practitioners. A central part of Kripalu's mission over the past ten years has been to host nonsectarian conversations among the many — and vastly different — spiritual and psychological traditions represented in this country. A compelling aspect of my job as scholar in residence has been to design and direct these conversations — often in the form of conferences or retreats. We have hosted numerous dialogues between Western-trained psychotherapists and yogis. We have sponsored conversations about spirit in the workplace, men's and women's spirituality, and nurturing the spirit in youth. And for the last four years, we have offered an annual conference on yoga and Buddhism, called East Meets East, at which most of the contributors to this volume have taught.

As part of each of these events, I have the opportunity, often on the last evening, to ask many senior American practitioners and teachers in the contemplative traditions to tell their stories. At the beginning of the evening, I pose my questions: "What inspired you to become involved in contemplative practice, and what continues to be your deepest source of inspiration? How has practice changed your life? What do you know about the teachings of your tradition, not through scripture, but through direct experience? What is the cutting edge of your personal practice? And finally, what do you believe is possible for you 'in this very life'?"

Since the very first of these retreats over ten years ago, I've noticed something interesting: In spite of all the fancy keynote talks and concurrent sessions we offer at these gatherings, students almost always feel most inspired by simply *hearing true stories of transformation — both the teachers' and their own.* As a result, I have learned to consistently plan these evening sessions when we just sit around as a group — as around a campfire — and listen to our stories of transformation. We have come to call these evenings "Tales from the Path."

This component of our gatherings has served to highlight a central theme of contemplative teaching: The most productive question that we can pose for ourselves is not "What can I know?" but "How should I live?" The problems with which the contemplative traditions wrestle are not primarily metaphysical. They are existential: "How might I live fully, completely, authentically?" Scriptures in both yoga and Buddhist traditions exhort practitioners to eschew metaphysics in favor of direct practice. "Perfection in yoga," says the *Hathayoga-Pradipika,* "is not achieved by wearing the apparel of a yogin, or by talking about it. Practice alone is the means to success. This is the truth, without doubt."

Many of us are increasingly familiar with the most important scriptures of these traditions: the *Yoga-sutra,* the *Hathayoga Pradipika,* the *Visuddhmagga,* the *Mahamudra,* the *Heart Sutra,* the *Diamond Sutra.* These scriptures are full of exotic descriptions of what it means to be a fully alive human being. They describe supernormal powers, highly concentrated mind states, deep forms of insight, and rapturous altered states of consciousness. These things, we know, are certainly possible for human beings. And this is compelling. But a quiet question emerges: What is possible for *me?* In this life? This year? Now?

This is the subject of one of Stephen Mitchell's most endearing poems, "Through the Eye of the Needle," a contemporary riff on the biblical parable of the camel and the needle.

The camel catches his breath, wipes the sweat from his brow. It was a tight squeeze, but he made it.

Lying back on the unbelievably lush grass, he remembers: all those years (how excruciating they were!) of fasting and one-pointed concentration, until finally he was thin enough: thauma-turgically thin, thread-thin, almost unrecognizable in his camelness: until the moment in front of his unblinking eye, when he put his front hooves together. Took one last breath. Aimed. Dived.

The exception may prove the rule, but what proves the exception? "It is not that such things are possible," the camel thinks, smiling. "But such things are possible for *me*."

Mitchell has here captured the central question of this book: What is possible for me? Not for the saints, the spiritual geniuses, those who can spend their lives in monasteries — but for me?

This, then, is the question I've posed to many of my friends and fellow yogis and meditators. In soliciting essays and interviews for this volume, I have asked each contributor to ponder three central questions:

1. **What do you believe is possible for you?** Sage Patanjali — author of the *Yoga-Sutra* — says that there are three ways of knowing: direct experience, inference, and the words of the masters. The first of these, he says — direct experience — is the form of knowing that leads to the most powerful kind of faith. This is sometimes called "verified faith." In what aspect of practice do you have "verified faith"? What do you know is possible from your direct experience.

2. It is said that one of the most important hallmarks of prac-

tice in the contemplative traditions is that it "bears fruit from the very beginning." Being as specific as you can, **what is the fruit that practice bears in your life?** What are the changes in your life that you believe to be deeply connected to practice in some fashion? The scriptures have many descriptions of the mature practitioner. But what does this maturity look like for you? Give us an "experience-near" picture of this ripening, if indeed ripening has taken place!

3. Finally, **what is the deepest source of your own inspiration?** Who or what is it that most inspires you, calls you out of yourself, has become a mirror in which you can see "the better angels of your nature"? If you'd like, give us one or two quotations from the most important source of your inspiration — a short statement whose words really draw you forward. I love the idea, articulated beautifully by Swami Ajaya, that we're drawn forward not from beneath, not by some instinctual life or the Freudian "drives," but rather pulled from above, by consciousness. What is it that tugs on you?

As you will see, these questions have yielded some fascinating stories. In looking at our contributors' essays as a collection, I've noticed, too, that most of them have addressed a question I did not actually ask, but one that hovers in the background of all American contemplative practice. What's possible for us in the context of this complex life we lead? In the context of this very worldly life? We are not monks, we say. We are not nuns, though on many days we might like to be. We are not able to decamp for long periods of time to a monastery in Southeast Asia or an ashram in India.

> "Each of the teachers and practitioners represented here has had to struggle with practice in the context of husbands, wives, children, aging parents, financial demands, illness and injury, grief, depressions, and neuroses of every imaginable kind."

One of the central challenges of contemplative practice in the West is that lay practitioners are engaging in highly esoteric practices that were often reserved in their cultures of origin for monks, nuns, wandering sadhus, and "renunciates" of all varieties. But how do these practices work in the context of our complicated lives "in the world"?

This volume of essays contains some fascinating answers to this question. Each of the teachers and practitioners represented here has had to struggle with practice in the context of husbands, wives, children, aging parents, financial demands, illness and injury, grief, depressions, and neuroses of every imaginable kind. And precisely in the context of these complex and difficult lives, we want to know: What difference has practice made?

Finally, I notice, too, that by bringing these stories together, we may have a beginning glimmer of an answer to another interesting question that I did not pose, but in which I've long been interested: We often ask how practice will change us. But what if we stand that question on its head? How will we change practice? How will these contemplative practices evolve and change through their contact with Western forms?

What happens when the "irresistible force" of practice meets the complexity of this historical moment? In America, traditional practice cultures have had to confront pluralism, democracy, feminism, allopathic medicine, gay men and lesbians, quantum physics, space exploration, New Age shamanism, and persons of all conceivable cultural and religious backgrounds. Clearly it is a time of great creativity and, perhaps, evolution in contemplative forms. Will they be diminished by their contact with us, or enhanced?

Early on in the transmission of the Eastern contemplative techniques to the West, Carl Jung warned that we should not take on these practices. He believed that they would too severely deconstruct the Western psyche. He warned that we should look instead to our own traditions, our own spiritual and psychological sources. Our experience over the last twenty-five years has shown us that Jung was clearly wrong for the most part. But he was right about one thing: We *will* need to find our own idiosyncratic paths into these traditions. We *will* have to make them ours. We *will* have to bring the principles alive with the stories of real American practice — the peculiar enigmas and conflicts of our twenty-first-century lives. We *will* need to respect our own cultures, psyches, and styles.

Heinrich Zimmer, one of the most articulate early students of the contemplative traditions, captured this truth on the very first page of his brilliant and groundbreaking book *The Philosophies of India:*

> We cannot take over the Indian solutions. We must enter the new period our own way and solve its questions for ourselves, because though truth, the radiance of reality, is universally one and the same, it is mirrored variously according to the mediums in which it is reflected. Truth appears differently in different lands and ages according to the living materials out of which its symbols are hewn.

Individual human beings are, of course, the "living materials" in which the truth is manifest, right here and right now. And it is precisely these dedicated individual practitioners who have become the doorways through which the contemplative traditions have entered American consciousness. Here, now, are their own Tales from the Path.

STEPHEN COPE
Lenox, Massachusetts
Summer 2003

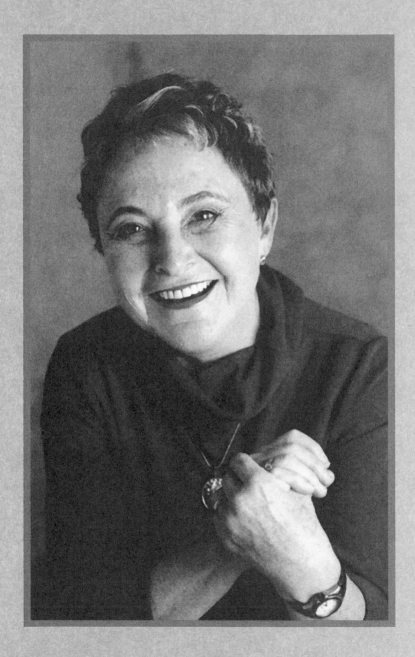

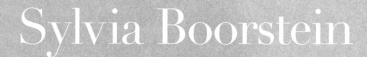

Sylvia Boorstein

I GOT KINDER

SYLVIA BOORSTEIN says about herself, "Whenever I fill out a form that asks for my occupation, I write 'teacher.' If I learn something useful, I look around for someone to tell it to." She began studying hatha yoga with Magana Baptiste in 1968 and began teaching it, with Magana's approval, in 1972. She has been a psychotherapist since 1967 and completed her doctorate in psychology in 1974. Her thesis title was "Hatha Yoga as a Very Gentle Psychotherapeutic Tool." • Sylvia began practicing Mindfulness meditation in 1977, and began to teach it in 1985. She has written four books on Buddhism and Mindfulness practice: *It's Easier Than You Think; Don't Just Do Something, Sit There; That's Funny, You Don't Look Buddhist;* and *Pay Attention, For Goodness' Sake.* • Sylvia is one of the founding teachers of Spirit Rock Meditation Center in Woodacre, California.

MY HUSBAND (whose spiritual practices are more intellectual, less contemplative than mine) and I have the following conversation periodically, motivated by nothing in particular, as part of breakfast-table conversation.

He: What do you think happened to you from all your years of meditation practice?

Me: I got kind.

He: You were *always* kind.

Me: I got *kinder.*

He: That's *it*? That's the whole thing?

Me: Essentially, that *is* it. But it has a fuller text, and footnotes. I can tell you more about it if you want to know.

Sometimes we talk further and sometimes we don't. I think his question truly isn't a challenge to prove something about meditation. He knows it has been tremendously beneficial to me. It's his way of saying affectionately, "I like you as much as I did fifty years ago, and for the same good reasons."

His question about the results of Mindfulness practice is an important one, though, to me, because clarity of intention — "Why am I doing this? Toward what end?" — is the primary determinant of how I practice and how I evaluate whether my practice is effective. As long as I am clear about what is *supposed* to happen, and by what mechanism it is supposed to happen, I'll be able to refine my practice, make it even more dedicated, more effective.

I began practicing Mindfulness twenty-five years ago, and it's apparent to me now that I had very little clarity of intention then.

This is why I started: I wanted to be less frightened. Although my teachers talked a lot about Enlightenment, which seemed mysterious and somewhat romantic, I didn't understand it well. When they described liberation as the absolute end of greed, hatred, and delusion and quoted scripture lines about the "plucking out of the defilements of the heart" so that they would never arise again — way beyond what I could imagine as possible for me — I didn't think seriously about whether I even *wanted* that to happen to me. I just wanted to be less frightened, less dreary in my thinking. I used to say, "I don't want to understand life. I just want to *stand* it." I assumed, in my fundamentally pragmatic style, that if Enlightenment — or even the path to Enlightenment — meant feeling better, it would include feeling less fearful.

> "My grandfather used to say, preceded by a great sigh, 'It's really hard to be a person!' It is."

I was forty years old. I had done all the things in life that I'd expected would be the causes of happiness — I'd been married for more than twenty years, I had four healthy, adolescent children, and I had a full-time professional life as a psychologist and, more recently, as a yoga teacher — and I was indeed grateful and happy for all of that. And/but, I was (still) basically anxious and mildly melancholic.

My demeanor is, by nature, cheerful, but I startle easily and I am easily overwhelmed. My sense of life, since early childhood, had been that it is difficult and unreliable, fraught with danger. I thought as my life became more and more complete in terms of what I could accomplish, my fearfulness would disappear. It didn't. When I encountered existential philosophy, in 1972, in graduate school — primarily reading Sartre and Kierkegaard and Camus — I found that it spoke directly to me. Among my family and friends I felt isolated in my melancholy, wished I were different, and imagined that meditation would make a difference.

I had also been — all of my life, although I am only beginning to admit it now — interested and excited by prayer. I did not quite know how to do devotional practice as a Jew. Judaism had been, and continues to be, what I think of as my religious path. But meditation practice, as I encountered it in Mindfulness retreats, seemed completely devout. *Quietly* devout, which is my style. I was immediately (and continue to be) contented by what I like to think of as "living in convent mode."

I liked hearing Dharma. I was consoled by the idea of the end of suffering long before I had any ability to calm or focus my attention. I remember the chagrin I felt when, after some significant period of practice, I realized that I had confused the promise of the end of suffering with the end of pain, which was what I *really* had hoped would happen. I was embarrassed not to have figured out something so obvious — really, what *could* I have been thinking?

Now I think of my vain hope for the end of all pain as a sweet example of how much I (maybe all of us) yearn to be more comfortable than we are. My grandfather used to say, preceded by a great sigh, "It's really hard to be a person!" It is. The Buddha said the same thing, more elegantly, in the First Noble Truth. Life is *dukkha,* unsatisfactory. The body needs continual care. Relationships need continual care. No matter how well you put things together, they don't stay that way. All of life, it turns out, is accommodating to changing conditions.

I was hoping to develop a different personality. I wanted what I imagined was a "spiritual style" in place of the style I had. I remember telling my teacher, Jack Kornfield, in an interview in the middle of a retreat, how dismayed I was by what I was increasingly witnessing, through my Mindfulness practice, about the tone of my psychological processes. "I'm so self-centered. Such a show-off! So extra dramatic! Hogging up conversations, having the last word, being such a raconteur! It is horrifying to me! I see it all so clearly! Being a Leo is not an excuse! I am stopping! After this retreat, you'll see. I will go home and be a different person. Diffident. Listening to other people's ideas. Not the center of conversations. Humble!"

Jack was very sweet. He listened. He said, "I don't know about that. I think we get issued one body and one personality for the trip."

I think that Jack is more or less right. I have the same body, only older, but recognizable as me. And I am still enjoying opportunities to tell people what I think. I think I'm toned down a little in flamboyance, less of a show-off perhaps, but I'm still dramatic. I'm not as self-conscious, though, about what I am as I was twenty-five years ago. I take my personality and talents and warts and all less seriously. I figure it is my karma, along with the genes for being short.

I did for a while have a glow-in-the-dark fantasy. I heard stories in the early years of my practice about amazing psychic talents that meditators developed, *siddhis,* like bi-location and levitation. And I remembered that I'd heard it said of my maternal grandmother that she glowed in the dark. I hoped I'd do that, too. When I began to be able to develop and sustain strong concentration states that included unusual and delightful manifestations of *piti,* or energy experiences in my body, I used to hope I was radiating light and that people would notice it. It was tantalizing to think about, but it didn't happen. Had it happened, it would have been its own problem.

Here is what actually happened from twenty-five years of practice, which definitely should be written as Work-in-Progress, since I am so (happily!) clear that it is a lifelong practice and that what has been happening will continue to happen, I hope cumulatively, for as long as I live.

I *am* kinder. I am kinder to myself and about myself, as well as kinder to other people. And the kindness has made me happier. Transformation happened along four parallel pathways. Here are the four paths, along with descriptions and vignettes of those paths.

●　　　●　　　●

I am kinder because I am more morally attentive. I see, faster than I used to, which habits of mine cause pain, to myself or to others, and I do them less because I know — I think we all do — that goodness creates happiness. Apart from people with very unusual and I think biologically unfortunate neurology, we don't take pleasure in being hurtful. We feel bad when we hurt someone, even accidentally. I feel better, if I realize I've caused pain, when I am able to ask forgiveness. "I am so sorry I did that. I intend not to do it again." I feel better making what amends I can, and feel reconnected with my own good intentions.

> "I am kinder. I am kinder to myself and about myself, as well as kinder to other people. And the kindness has made me happier."

It has been my experience that nothing is ever lost from the moral inventory file. My first clear experience of this was on retreat, many years ago. Suddenly, in the midst of feeling wonderful, my mind began what felt like a computer readout of every mean-spirited thing I had ever done. I was dismayed, not to speak of humiliated. I said to my teacher, "I have done something wrong!" She said, "No. You've done it right. This is, after all, called the Path of Purification of the Heart."

I think it is completely true for me to say, now, that I welcome this predictable, spontaneous readout, on retreat and off as well. I enjoy thinking of practice as the Path of Purification. I feel better when I am untroubled by conscience. The Buddha called a clear conscience the Bliss of Blamelessness — and I find it to be a full-time job. "Oh dear, why did I end that phone conversation so suddenly? She needed to talk just a little bit more, and I got restless . . ." Or, "I shouldn't have said that. That probably hurt her feelings."

I recall hearing early on in my meditation practice: "People who achieve the first particular identifiable level of direct understanding are unable to break a precept!" I understood that to mean that those people are never again able to harm living beings, or take anything at all not freely given, or express their sexuality in any way that is exploitive or abusive, or speak at all in a way that causes pain, and that they are committed to never confusing the mind with intoxicants of any sort.

What is true for me now is that although I am more careful than ever to pay attention to my actions, I still make mistakes. My conscience catches up with me faster than it used to, though, so it's a kindness to myself to get it right the first time. And it is also a kindness to myself not to struggle with guilt. When I do make mistakes, when I cause pain, I am less hard on myself than I used to be — "Whoops. Made a mistake. Clean it up. Make the phone call now. Apologize." — because I know I am doing the best I can, and that my intention is goodness. I make allowances for myself for having been tired, or confused, or overwhelmed in any of the ways in which human beings are overwhelmed.

●　　●　　●

I am kinder because I am calmer and less fearful. I have echoes of my former anxieties, but I am not held hostage by them. I still startle, but not as much. I am less easily confused, and so more naturally good-hearted (more kind) more of the time. I think my neurology changed. I believe that the periods of time that I have spent in deep states of concentration, states developed through both Mindfulness practice and Lovingkindness practice, were very important.

I once asked my friend and teacher, Jack Kornfield, "When did I start to change, really?" He said, "You were changing all along, from the beginning, but the most incremental change happened when you started your *Metta* (Lovingkindness) practice."

I like to think of my concentration practice as being the catalyst that moved my understanding from thinking that Dharma was true to knowing it deeply in the fiber of my being.

A most dramatic example of changed neurology happened not long ago when the flight I was on, returning to San Francisco, flew into a storm of such intensity that the flight crew needed to stay in their seats for an hour and all the passengers on the flight closed their laptops, put away reading material, tightened their seat belts, and braced themselves. It was night, so the view out the window was all blackness. Although I've never really liked flying, and this lurching and bumping flight was the wildest I'd ever been on, I felt at ease. I thought, "This is new! Who could have imagined this as a possibility?" I was happy. I turned to the man sitting next to me and asked, "How are you?"

"I'm fine," he replied.

We'd had some conversation earlier and I knew he flew a lot as part of his work.

"This is an unusually rough ride, isn't it?" I asked.

"Yeah," he said. "It is. But, you know, I figure that when your number is up, it's up. Everyone dies sometime."

I thought about how he might have been the Buddha, talking about *anicca,* impermanence, and how the insight of impermanence — the insight that we hope to experience so profoundly in meditation that it becomes cellular, visceral, in our response pattern — seemed to be firmly established in him. Things change. Everything dies. It's out of anyone's control. Everyone really knows that, I thought, but some people don't get startled out of remembering. I was having a good time. Imagine. After a lifetime of vaguely anxious if not worried flying, all of a sudden it was seeming to me like Disneyland and I was having a good time — an *especially* good time because I wasn't frightened. It seemed like a miracle.

I've spent lots of time in my life "explaining" my easily worrying mind. I've hypothesized that my anxiety might be a consequence of my mother's frail health when I was a child, my own poor health during my childhood, my frequent illnesses, and my long absences from school. Sometimes, if I pay attention to my dreams, I think it is racial, part of tribal memory. More recently I think it is genetic, a reflection of my neurology, or my past karma, which would also contribute to my neurology. Maybe it is all of the above. The etiology of my easily worrying mind is not as important to me now as it used to be. What matters to me is that I am changed!

The plane shook and lurched this way and that. I waited to get nervous and it didn't happen. I kept up my conversation with the man next to me and the woman next to him. All the while I talked I could hear the *Metta* chant I do as habit playing itself in my mind, alternating with my chant of Psalm 117, my alternative concentration practice. We told stories of other bumpy flights we had taken, I think to amuse and support each other. We all knew it was an uncommonly rough flight. I liked the fact that we three were caring for each other, doing the kindness of keeping each other company. I loved it that I could be a part of it.

It was what I could not have imagined twenty-five years ago would be a result of my practice: being able to do my life as it happens, being able to say, "It's like this," acknowledging the truth of what's happening, recognizing when I can, or cannot, do anything about it, and not struggling with it. I am hugely reassured when I see that it is happening. Sitting in the plane, bumping along, enjoying not being anxious, I thought that the difference between that flight and other flights before, and perhaps other flights yet to come, was that my mind was really balanced. I thought it was probably — but not completely — the result of having been away teaching, and doing a lot of meditation practice. I also thought, "Maybe I'm actually getting wiser!"

●   ●   ●

SYLVIA BOORSTEIN

I am kinder because I am less opinionated. I used to say that I was opinionated because I came from a long line of opinionated women. Now I think it had more to do with being afraid I didn't know the "right" answer. Being less frightened allows me to be less opinionated, less wedded to views, more tolerant, more able to consider that the other person might be right and I could be wrong. I still have views. It's not about having, or not having, views. It's about not being attached to them. For me, giving up the need to know the right answer all the time is either considerable psychological growth or a deep understanding of emptiness, the knowing and actually experiencing that there is no one whose ego needs to be protected. I think it's both. My psyche got a little more healed and my soul woke up a little.

> "I am determined not to be an enemy to anyone. Having enemies is an unkindness to myself."

Here is one more story: I recently had what amounted to the third rage attack of my life. A project that I had wanted to do, one that I worked for several months to get organized and in place, was not going to happen because someone else, whose cooperation was required, decided at the last minute not to go along with it. I pleaded my cause but I did not prevail. I was angry, and by the time I arrived home, obsessively thinking about it, I was enraged. I come from mild-mannered people and I am generally mild-mannered. Wrath felt awful. It invaded my mind like a demon. It took some days for it to die down, and some time after that to work out a compromise agreement.

Even as the experience was unfolding, however, I was aware of not having made the other person "my enemy." I was dismayed, certainly challenged, and wanting very much to have "my way" happen, but I also was aware of thinking quite soon, "This other person is not my enemy, and what's more, this person might be right. I don't think so, but maybe." In the end, I'm not sure whether my way, or that person's way, or the compromise way, was the "best" way. Who knows, really? The immediate results of any project are not the final results. Things get set in motion, and then other things happen, and then others. Admitting "I didn't know" kept the other person off my enemy list, and a "No Enemy List" is a most important part of how I think about my practice right now. I understand the meditation phrase that I use for concentration, "May I be free of enmity and danger," as meaning free of my own enmity. I am determined not to be an enemy to anyone. Having enemies is an unkindness to myself.

•   •   •

I am kinder because I am more zealous than ever about social activism. I see my activism as an aspect of spiritual practice, the natural result of being less frightened, as well as a sign of liberated energy available for purposes other than just keeping myself going. However much I gravitate to retreat spaces and love them, I am more ardent than ever about sharing the practice of peace with the world. It's the increased ardency that is new. I always thought that spiritual practice was a part of regular life, and that social activism was obligatory. I grew up in a traditionally observant Jewish family whose religious heart expressed itself in support of liberal politics, labor unionizing in the early part of the twentieth century, and civil rights. Voting, in my family, was a religious act. I am very happy when I feel I am being helpful.

> "I look at the world now, suffering as it is, and more than ever I understand that I cannot end greed, hatred, and delusion in anyone but myself."

A commentary that follows the Buddha's Sermon on the Foundations of Mindfulness is called Clear Comprehension of Purpose, and it calls in various ways for staying, in modern language, "on task." I look at the world now, suffering as it is, and more than ever I understand that I cannot end greed, hatred, and delusion in anyone but myself. But in those brief moments in which I sense them to be absent in me, I think "It is for this moment that I have been practicing. I am free. I am not frightened. I am not humiliated by guilt. I really am in love with all beings and with the world and with life, and I am able to serve." ●

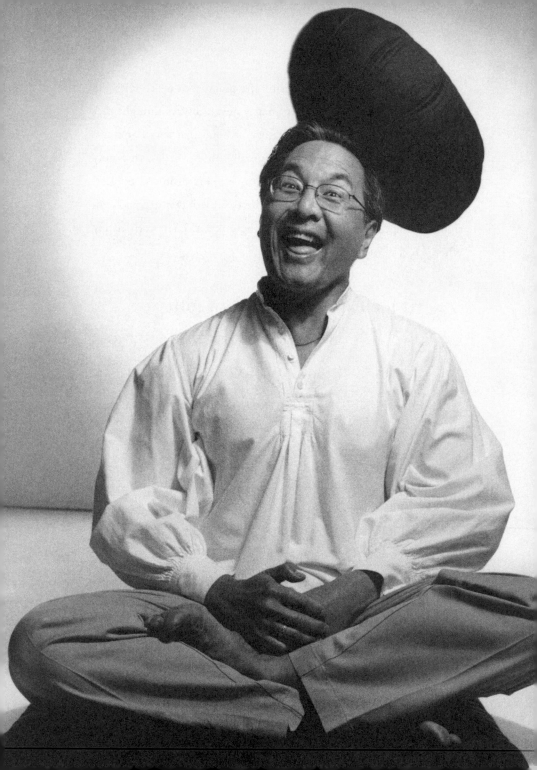

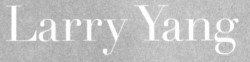

Larry Yang

LARRY YANG, LCSW, feels grateful that he has had the opportunity to reincarnate more than once in this lifetime. A psychotherapist and most recently clinical supervisor and program coordinator for Diversity and Multicultural Services at San Francisco General Hospital's outpatient psychotherapy clinic, Larry is also a consultant and trainer on multicultural issues from a perspective of contemplative and spiritual practice. His articles "Directing the Mind Towards Practices in Diversity" and "Metta as Diversity Practice" were included in *Friends on the Path: Living Spiritual Communities,* by Thich Nhat Hanh. Larry is a coeditor of *Making the Invisible Visible: Healing Racism in Our Buddhist Communities.* As a gay man of color training in the Theravadan Buddhist tradition, he is part of the Community Dharma Leaders and Dedicated Practitioners Programs of Spirit Rock Meditation Center and is on their Diversity Council. • In the past, Larry was a graphic designer trained in the master of fine arts program at Yale University. His design work is in the Cooper-Hewitt Museum, Metropolitan Museum of Fine Art, and Museum of Modern Art. Prior to that, Larry was a park ranger for the National Park Service in southern Utah and northern California. • Indications are that another incarnation is emerging.

WITHIN THE IRREVERENT NATURE of gay/queer vernacular language, I might be considered a "process queen" — a person who is more focused on the process of a task than on the outcome itself. I am drawn to examining questions before attempting answers. So when I'm asked, "Have the practices of yoga and meditation changed your life?" I find myself restructuring the question. My experience is that everything changes my life — every expansive and minute experience of joy or pain or boredom. Everything changes my life; thus — yes, yoga and meditation have changed my life. It is also true in my experience that life changes . . . with or without yoga or meditation.

Life changes with or without my intervention, interference, or influence. There are times when I look at aged photographs of myself as a sleepy Chinese tot, wrapped in cotton blankets patterned with designs of dancing alphabets and singing animals, and I am awestruck at how life has changed from then until now.

Gazing into the sky of a 1963 midsummer day, a solitary eight-year-old Chinese boy plays a universal game of creating shapes and objects and beings out of the ever-shifting wisps of white clouds traveling from horizon to horizon. The innocence of that boy's gaze belies the life that was changed as he was repeatedly called words that diminished and caricatured his cultural background by other children who were beginning to learn the methods of an often unequal and unjust society. Life certainly changed.

During that time I felt a deep connection to my family's generational tree as my mother would tell stories of our family's life before immigration — including how my mother's father believed in the education of women when it was unheard of in Chinese culture, or how my father's family placed all their resources (and I mean *all* their resources) into my father's education as the firstborn son in order to lift him from their ancestral rural village to the dream of some unknown but hope-filled potential. She would tell her stories over green tea and sunflower seeds, sharing the deep values and cultural meanings of the Middle Path with her Western-born son.

However, the world in those years never felt completely safe. There were those other stories of dark-suited FBI agents coming to our house when my father was at work, and stories of my mother being interrogated for receiving Chinese language newspapers during the years of Joseph McCarthy. There was the story of my father's realization that over many years as a college professor he was being paid consistently less than his Caucasian peers. There were my own tales of childhood: of being ostracized by kids from whom I looked different, and of always hiding another secret from everyone else — of being a boy who felt the need for more connection and relationship with other boys.

In the balance of things, even with hindsight, life usually felt more painful than not. Along with the obsession to escape such pain, I became determined to become that which I was not. I lost interest in my language of origin, my cultural heritage, and the deep sources of my identity. Family history and lineage became quaint stories that I tolerated to humor my parents and relatives over holidays, but which did not concern me in my "real life."

I measured myself against the achievements of others who looked as if they belonged to the American mainstream, those who seemed successful in the dominant culture. I wanted to assimilate without conditions. Instead of feeling separation, I craved connection and the feeling that I belonged, hoping to escape the pain that I knew to exist. In a determined exertion of willpower, I remember having the fixed conviction that "if it is this difficult to be a person of color, there is no way that I will be gay" — adding another lock to the closet door.

I recall that as a "business person" — a person in a serious business of climbing ladders while looking nonchalant — the slogan of my firm was "The Only Constant Is Change." Little did I know that we were unintentionally tapping into the deepest wisdom of the nature of things: impermanence.

Ultimately, because I had a lot of un-wisdom at the time, the irony was on me, because a time arrived when the materialism that gave me pleasure, inspiration, and joy . . . no longer did. My attempts at assimilation into a heterosexual white culture took me further away from my identity as a gay Chinese man. This gap between realities became deeper as the contradiction continued. The void was filled repeatedly with unending and excessive amounts of alcohol, drugs, caffeine, and nicotine — anything but the real feelings of the experience. Perhaps I hoped the void would somehow be soothed or fixed by not feeling anything at all.

And life changed.

Was it due to luck? Circumstance? Karma? All that I know is that the force with which life changes is immense.

When I came to spiritual practice, I had already done some letting go — enough at least to know that I did not know anything, especially about life. With that perspective, practice supported me. Practice supported me, not in giving me skills in understanding and controlling life, but rather in teaching me how to relate to it. And now, finally, to answer the original question: Practice may have changed my life, but I have benefited most by the offer from my practice to experience life fully as it changes. Practice has changed my relationship to the unfolding stories of my life.

The moment-to-moment nature of contemplative awareness, observation, inquiry, and reflection, through all experiences of joy, pain, and boredom, has changed my relationship to each. When stories of separation or oppression are triggered or re-created, there is a new curiosity about the deepest nature of my experience. This curiosity allows spaciousness to enter the suffering. Experiences of joy are held with a new sense of value and respect, knowing that, as stories, they too will change and lead necessarily to other events.

As I sit in meditation or hold an asana, the awareness of the nature of my reality (as much as I can intuit and discern) is a template for my overall experience. The recognition that even the easiest yoga postures create discomfort over time — and that the most comfortable sitting positions create suffering — has revealed how I might hold the twists and turns of the mental and emotional asanas that emerge moment to moment. The micro-opportunities to let go and become more aware in a physical pose have helped me unravel the mental contortions that happen in my mind.

Likewise, in meditation, noting sensation after sensation — not needing to become involved in the sensations or to interpret them, but simply to be aware — strengthens my awareness, and I experience a growing capacity to let go of each sensation as a new one arises. Letting go of the previous sensation allows the next sensation to emerge. Holding on to the previous sensation creates obstructions to experiencing the next moment fully. Holding on to previous moments becomes living in the past, even if for a few microseconds; anticipating the next moment becomes living in the future.

When there is a letting go, there is permission for the present experience to fill my awareness fully. There is a peace and ease of mind regardless of the circumstance or story that I am living. And as my mind begins to ease, so does my life. Amazing . . . that it is so simple, but of course it's not so easy to execute.

Last fall I was rushing to meet a friend for dinner and had to get some cash from the ATM that I always use near my home in San Francisco. I waited impatiently and unmindfully for my turn, and when I reached to insert my card, I stopped abruptly. My awareness became sharp as a knife. Scratched into different areas of the ATM faceplate were the words: "Chinese Garbage," "Chinese Trash," "Chinese Shit."

The film of the scene that I was living shifted into slow motion. Dinner plans suddenly became a distraction and my focus telescoped into "What is happening right now? What is my internal experience?" The rush of pressure to my head, the pounding of increased blood circulation, a dizziness and detachment from my surroundings were immediately identifiable. As I tuned in to the detachment, I felt aversion and the desire to escape, to push away the present moment. That which *was,* I did not *want* to be.

As I lifted the veil of aversion and anger, there was revealed a tremendous sadness that was felt by an eight-year-old boy who had his head in the clouds. I began to see the elderly Asian couples walking by me — barely supporting each other in their frailty — as my mother and father. I felt my heart embrace their experience and what their responses might be to this disparagement of their identity. I saw others passing by as versions of myself or akin to me as brother or sister, and I felt their injuries. But I also felt the injury of the injurer — how the perpetrator must have been deeply wounded in order to create such a harmful event for others. From this deliberate expansion in examining my current experience came the realization that the eight-year-old boy's relationship to such events had changed. Life had changed.

Sometime later I was sitting at the table after dinner with my mother and father, now in their late eighties, along with my partner of several years (another example of how life changes). Over green tea and sunflower seeds, I was explaining to them aspects of my livelihood in supervising and training cultural competency at a psychotherapy clinic, as well as aspects of my spiritual practice in developing diversity trainings using contemplative and mindfulness practices. They were clearly engaged and intent upon my words, nodding and responding with attentiveness, though there was little actual discussion.

In the quiet space that followed, I felt the dynamic interplay of complex feelings in the room: pride in the person their son turned out to be; sadness that their son turned out to be so different from them; concern for risks that he takes in an adverse society; wondering if they had made mistakes in his parenting; questioning how Western versus Chinese he had become, yet pleased that he was of both cultures; ambivalence and conflicted feelings about his orientation; and not knowing what was the "right" thing to say.

I found myself responding with a similar silence, holding the space and absorbing all the feelings in the room. I no longer needed to react by defending my decisions, or lifestyle, or opinions. I could allow all of their experience to interplay with all of mine, without adding any other energy.

The following week was my birthday and I received a card from them. On the front of the card, it read: "You make our family tree . . . "

I opened the card: " . . . a lot more interesting."

It was signed "We love you, Mom and Dad"

To my mother and father: You are as much a part of my spiritual practice as any yoga or meditation, and my yoga and meditation practice has helped me to become aware of that. I love you, too. ●

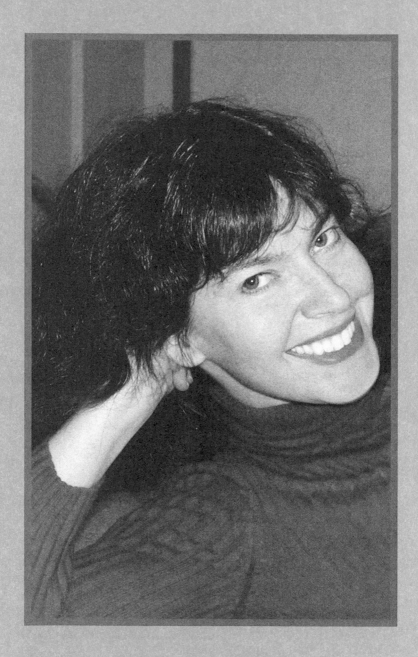

Anne Cushman

LIVING FROM THE INSIDE OUT

ANNE CUSHMAN grew up as a "military brat" on Army posts from Kansas to Korea. After surviving three years in a Connecticut boarding school, she went on to Princeton University, where she majored in comparative religion and began exploring Eastern contemplative practices. Her senior thesis — a video documentary about a Los Angeles Zen center and its teacher — turned into a groundbreaking investigation of a spiritual community in crisis, which grounded her idealism in the reality of human frailties. • After falling in love with hatha yoga, Anne trained as a yoga teacher and became an editor for *Yoga Journal,* while continuing to study and practice Buddhist meditation. She has studied with, interviewed, and written about many of the most powerful and innovative teachers of our time, both Eastern and Western. She traveled to India to research the roots of yoga and Buddhism, an investigation that resulted in her spiritual guidebook, *From Here to Nirvana.* • A contributing editor to both *Yoga Journal and Tricycle: The Buddhist Review,* Anne now lives with her three-year-old son, Skye, in Marin County, California, where she teaches yoga at Spirit Rock Meditation Center and writes about the intersection of spiritual practice with the grit and chaos of everyday life.

I FELL IN LOVE WITH YOGA sixteen years ago when I was twenty-three. I was living with two massage students in an adobe cabin on the southern border of Santa Fe, New Mexico, out where the art galleries and million-dollar villas disintegrated into a tattered fringe of vacant lots and trailer home parks. Our cabin smelled of mouse droppings, a comforting smell reminiscent of the gerbil cages in second-grade classrooms. It had a woodstove in the kitchen, and an abandoned chicken coop in the yard, and an enormous tepee out by the woodpile, where my roommates and I used to gather to bang on congas and rattle gourds while incanting visualizations of our futures. "If it's for my highest good," we'd begin, "I create a reality in which . . . " There was always a certain amount of anxiety in these prayers, as if God were a moody and unpredictable waitress, and if we forgot to mention that we wanted cream in our coffee or a lover who wasn't already secretly married, there would be no chance to change our order.

It was my roommate Lori who took me to my first yoga class, taught in the early morning at her massage school by one of the students, a slender man with muscles so clearly defined that the massage teacher used to strip him to his underwear and use him as an animated anatomy text. My main reason for going, frankly, was that I couldn't afford to get Rolfed. I'd been reading about Rolfing in one of my roommate's massage manuals: how your skeleton could be popped apart like a two-year-old's Barbie doll and put back together in better alignment. I longed to be remade like that — a fresh start, from the bones up, like having your engine rebuilt by God. But

Rolfing was sixty dollars a session, way more than I could afford on my five-dollar-an-hour check for my part-time job as a product tester for an interactive video company. So I decided to try yoga instead.

The carpeted room smelled of almond body oil, sweat, and steaming brown rice. The teacher stood at the front of the room in threadbare gray sweatpants, naked from the waist up. As he swung his arms overhead in a Sun Salutation, slabs of muscles slid around his chest and back; then he folded in two at the hips. I took a deep breath and dove in.

> "For the first time, I was feeling my own body from the inside, swimming in a swirling stream of sensations. After years of trying to *watch* my breath, finally I was *being* it."

At twenty-three I wasn't a newcomer to Eastern spiritual practices. Two years earlier I had graduated from Princeton University with a degree in comparative religion, concentrating on Buddhism and Hinduism. I had spent months in my dingy basement carrel at Firestone Library, in the flickering, greenish glow of fluorescent lights, drinking metallic decaf from a vending machine and taking notes on texts that told me Buddhism couldn't be found in books. For my senior thesis, I'd gotten a National Endowment for the

Humanities grant to produce a documentary about Zen in America, and had spent a month at the Zen Center of Los Angeles with my filmmaker boyfriend, videotaping interviews with teachers and practitioners. I'd started an intermittent meditation practice, sat a couple of Zen *sesshins,* and begun thinking of myself as a Buddhist.

But as I folded, arched, breathed, and sweated through that first yoga practice in Santa Fe, I could feel that something different was starting to happen. My body thrummed like a plucked guitar string. Energy buzzed and tingled in my spine. I could feel my breath pulse through my whole body — rippling my vertebrae, spreading my ribs, sending waves of sensation through bones and muscles and organs and skin.

Meditation, for me, had always been a cerebral experience, with "me" sitting firmly in my own head, observing my breath and body (that itchy nostril! that stabbing knee!) like a theater critic reviewing a particularly maddening play. But now, for the first time, I was feeling my own body from the inside, swimming in a swirling stream of sensations. After years of trying to *watch* my breath, finally I was *being* it.

It reminded me of one of my recurring dreams: that a wall in my house had lifted up and revealed a whole other room — magical, mysterious — that I hadn't even known was there.

From that moment forward, hatha yoga and Buddhist meditation have always flowed together for me. On Vipassana retreats in California and New Mexico — my hips throbbing and my neck pinched from long hours of cross-legged sitting — I'd duck out of walking meditation to do Sun Salutations amid the pine trees and yuccas. On retreats at Plum Village, the French community of Vietnamese Zen master Thich Nhat Hanh, I'd get up at dawn to stand on my head on the dewy grass outside my tent, while the sun rose over fields of sunflowers. As I sat in meditation, I'd feel the tingle and pulse of the energy I'd awakened through yoga postures. And at the heart of a sweaty yoga practice, I could rest in the stillness I'd cultivated while I sat on my cushion.

> "Moving my body into different shapes,
> I became a different person.
> Creating more space in my joints, I made
> more space in my mind as well."

These yoga breaks always felt a little illicit, as though I was sneaking out of the meditation retreat to have a margarita and get laid. In those days, most hard-core Buddhist practitioners looked down on yoga as excessively sensual and body-obsessed — after all, how could you take seriously a spiritual practice that was performed in pink Lycra tights? The Buddha, they pointed out, had studied with the greatest yogis of India, but rejected their body-based practices as too extreme and ultimately ineffective at bringing about lasting happiness. And in contemporary Western culture — at a time when "yoga" is associated, in the popular consciousness, with sleek young actresses flexing in skintight unitards on Gucci yoga mats — it's all too easy to get attached to the glittering goals of the sculpted buttocks and pectorals, or the head arched back to the soles of the feet in a perfect King Cobra. All of these forms are impermanent, my Buddhist teachers reminded me; all of them will die and rot.

But I kept on doing yoga — because I found that for me, there was no faster way to transform my mind than to move my body. Yoga offered me a direct access to a kind of joy that arose straight from my nerves and bones, independent of external circumstances. In Western terms, this transformation can be described in terms of hormones and nerve synapses and endorphins; in Eastern terms, it's a function of *prana* and chakras and energies flowing through a network of subtle channels. In either case, the experience was the same — a transformation of all the subjective sensations that gave rise to my sense of self. Moving my body into different shapes, I became a different person. Creating more space in my joints, I made more space in my mind as well. Twisting and bending and arching my body, I broke up the ice floes of self-judgment that had frozen in my muscles. I squeezed out the anxiety knotted between my shoulder blades. I melted the anger in the pit of my stomach into tears.

I may come to my mat miserable, tense, constricted, burdened by judgments of all the things that I'm not that I should be and all the things that I should be that I'm not. The walls of my mind close in on me like a trash compactor. "You haven't accomplished enough," jeer the voices in my head, "and what you have accomplished is not any good." But at the end of the practice, I'll leave the mat with every cell of my body singing with pleasure and my heart wide open. My inner hecklers hurl their taunts and tomatoes from a distant corner of my mind, their voices irrelevant, almost inaudible.

•   •   •

Almost ten years ago, I made a pilgrimage to India to visit the places associated with the Buddha's life. I explored the buried ruins of monasteries marking the site of the palace in Nepal where the young Siddhartha was raised as a prince in the Sakya clan. I hiked up a heat-baked hill to meditate in the tiny, smoke-blackened cave where Siddhartha had spent six years in ascetic practice, starving himself until his spine showed through the skin of his belly and his buttocks looked like horses' hooves. I walked on the banks of the river where he renounced asceticism and ate the rice pudding offered to him by a village girl.

> "Yoga grounds my awareness, again
> and again, in cartilage, muscle,
> organs, and bone; it hooks me back into
> the moment-to-moment unfolding
> of embodied experience."

I meditated beneath the branches and heart-shaped leaves of the *bodhi tree* — a fourth-generation descendant of the actual tree that sheltered the Buddha as he attained enlightenment — and listened to the sonorous chanting of hundreds of Tibetan monks, deep and unfathomable as the mind itself. As tinny music jangled from a chairlift across the valley, I watched a magenta sunset from Vulture Peak, where the Buddha first preached the Heart Sutra, proclaiming that "form is emptiness, emptiness is form." As lemur monkeys quarreled in the sal trees overhead, I circumambulated a stupa in Kushinagar that commemorates the place where he died of food poisoning in his eighties.

My trip to India brought home for me a very simple truth: The Buddha was a human being, in a human body. Like any other person, he was born, walked on the earth, and died. And his great awakening took place in this body — indeed, *through* this body — a body that, like anyone else's, got sick, got hungry, shat, pissed, fell apart.

After all, most of the experiences that I think of as most spiritual — being born, giving birth, loving another person, losing loved ones to death, dying myself — are also intensely physical, irrevocably entwined with the messy, sensual business of blood and nerves and skin.

Yoga grounds my awareness, again and again, in cartilage, muscle, organs, and bone; it hooks me back into the moment-to-moment unfolding of embodied experience, which at other times I am all too willing to ignore in favor of the alluring fantasies spun by my mind. My practice reminds me that the specifics of my physical experience in this moment — this belly full of French toast, this pelvis skewed slightly to the right from carrying a baby on my hip all morning, this tangible sorrow shrink-wrapped around my heart — are the doorway into the infinite, the place where I touch the whole of creation. As I explore the wilderness of my own body, I see that I am made of blood and bones, sunlight and water, pesticide residues and redwood humus, the fears and dreams of generations of ancestors, particles of exploded stars.

Whether you call it genes or karma, my body carries with it the encoded stories of lifetime after lifetime. I've got the fair freckled skin and racehorse nerves of my Irish ancestors, the tight jaw and stern willpower of my Puritan ones. Opening into a back bend, I touch my grandmother's grief — lodged deep in my own heart — for a child dead at age four. Surrendering into a forward bend, I meet the resistance of what my chiropractor calls my military neck — passed down from my father the army general, and his father the army general, who stood tall and swallowed their fear.

Yoga encourages me to focus my awareness with exquisite precision — to feel into the space between two thoracic vertebrae; to sense the skin on the inner armpit; to notice the flickers of joy and sorrow alternating with every heartbeat. And then — on a good day — I can begin to see the rest of my life with that kind of poet's precision. My practice can remind me to bow down to all the intimate, ordinary details of my life — whether I'm picking smashed raisins from the floor by my son's highchair or clicking on Netscape to open my e-mail — with that same sort of tender appreciation, like an artist painting an apple over and over again, worshipping it with her brush.

•   •   •

When I started doing yoga, I actually thought there was somewhere to get. Shuffling through old files recently, I found a yoga exam from my days in a teacher-training program at the Iyengar Yoga Institute in San Francisco, in which the teacher had asked us to describe four poses that we found difficult, and to describe what we were going to do to master them. Earnestly, I described my challenges — the tight hips in Revolved Triangle Pose, the tucked-under sitting bones in Seated Forward Bend — and outlined the steps I was taking to eradicate them. Implicit in my answer was the belief that my challenges were both finite and soluble, that with diligent practice I would root them out and arrive at perfection.

In those days I still thought that "doing things right" was the point of yoga. In my mind my life stretched ahead of me as an endless upward spiral. Through my practice, I imagined, I'd root out all my messy imperfections: my tight hamstrings, my rambling mind, my possessiveness and jealousy, the way my left shoulder lifted higher than the right. Like my Downward Dog Pose, my whole life would come into perfect alignment. I'd learn to sing on key. I'd write a best-selling novel. I'd revel in public speaking. I'd only fall in love with people who fell in love with me.

Nowadays, my practice is different. My body has not gotten better and better, like an upgrading software program. Instead, despite my best efforts, it's wearing out, breaking down, growing softer and looser and weaker. In the last ten years I've lugged a backpack all over India. I've twisted a knee jogging and pulled a muscle doing the splits and thrown my back out moving boxes of books.

I've cut back on yoga practice to write a book. I've carried two babies to term. These days I can't do back bends I used to do effortlessly. Kicking up into an Elbow Balance the other day, I toppled over with a graceless thud. One day in yoga class, after being up and down all night with my teething one-year-old, I actually fell asleep in a Shoulder Stand.

> "These days, my practice is teaching me to embrace imperfection: to have compassion for all the ways things haven't turned out as I planned, in my body and in my life — for the way things keep falling apart, and failing, and breaking down."

These days, my practice is teaching me to embrace imperfection: to have compassion for all the ways things haven't turned out as I planned, in my body and in my life — for the way things keep falling apart, and failing, and breaking down. It's less about fixing things, and more about learning to be present for exactly what is.

My yoga practice has helped me be present through the terrible loss of delivering my stillborn daughter, Sierra, and the almost unbearable joy of receiving my newborn son Skye in my arms, wet and wide-eyed and lifting his wobbly head to turn toward his daddy's voice. It's taught me to begin to embrace my body and my life in all their ragged edges and cellulite: to open to a neck that goes out and a friend who lets me down and muscles that won't let go and a child who won't sleep through the night. It reminds me how futile are all my attempts to control my body and my life, and that when it comes right down to it, I can't control or hang onto anything that's really important.

But it also reminds me that despite all this — or perhaps because of this — my life is precious and glorious. It's teaching me to find some sort of balance and ease in the uncertainty, as though I'm doing a handstand poised at the edge of a cliff.

When I do yoga these days, I feel like one of those yogis I used to see in India doing a headstand in the center of a circle of fire, or sitting in lotus by a funeral pyre on the banks of the Ganges, watching a body burn. I know the world is in flames all around me, I know my body is on its way back to the earth. But in the middle of it all, I can breathe and stretch and flow and dance; I can reach my arms to the sky, and bow my head to the earth, and feel my body ringing like a temple bell.

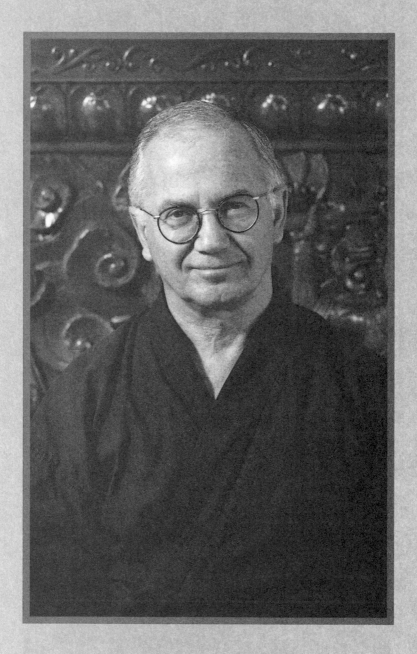

Larry Rosenberg

TASTING THE SILENCE

LARRY ROSENBERG has a Ph.D. in social psychology from the University of Chicago. He taught and did research at Harvard Medical School, the University of Chicago, and Brandeis University before leaving academic life to train in Dharma. His first teacher was J. Krishnamurti, with whom he studied until Krishnamurti's death in 1986. • Larry spent years in the study and practice of hatha yoga, Vedanta, as well as Zen and Vipassana. He has studied with masters in India, Japan, Korea, Thailand, and America. The focus of Larry's study for more than twenty years has been Vipassana meditation in the Theravadan tradition. He is currently a guiding teacher at Cambridge Insight Meditation Center in Cambridge, Massachusetts, and a teacher at Insight Meditation Society in Barre, Massachusetts. • Larry's publications include *Breath by Breath: The Liberating Practice of Insight Meditation* and *Living in the Light of Death: On the Art of Being Truly Alive.*

Q. *Have yoga and meditation really changed your life, Larry?*

A. Well, my parents had an interesting perspective on that question that I'd like to share. My parents, who are Russian-Jewish immigrants, came to Cambridge Insight Meditation Center once to hear me teach, and I gave a dharma talk to a hall full of people. At the end of it someone turned to my parents and said: "Mr. and Mrs. Rosenberg, you've known Larry all his life. Has meditation actually improved him?" My mother jumped to her feet, irate, and with her thick accent she said: "Improve him? Improve him? He never needed any improvement." I was embarrassed, to put it mildly! But of course I think it has helped me. In fact it's transformed me in many ways.

Q. *Can you say what some of those ways are?*

A. I have more energy now, and a different kind of energy. I taught for ten years as a professor. It felt that I was on the line a lot; it was tiring — not in a "good honest work" way, but rather as though there was too much at stake while I was teaching. I worried about what people would think of what I had to say.

The turning point for me came in my first year of teaching at Harvard. I had incredibly unrealistic projections about what it would do for me. My father was a cab driver, and here I was a Harvard professor. I expected the job would end my anxieties, would fix everything. It didn't fix anything. My ego felt terrific and

I had money for the first time in my life, but at a certain point I got depressed. I realized this wasn't Harvard's fault. I was depressed because I had wanted this to transform me. It didn't, and that's what got me to look inside. Up to that point I was still looking for happiness externally. Out of my depression grew a realization that I was looking in the wrong place.

Q. *Why do you say you have more energy now, and of a different kind?*

A. I think part of why I have more energy now, even though I work just as hard or harder, is that — I can't say that I'm ego-less, that would be extravagant — but I'm not using dharma teaching to puff up my ego/identity. I'm concerned with carrying out the function of teaching as best I can, but I don't feel there's so much riding on it. I don't build status out of it.

Practice has helped me in other ways, too. I had a tremendous fear of aging and death. So a teacher named Ajaan Suwat, from the Thai Forest (Kammatthana) tradition, put me through some pretty rigorous classical Buddhist training on aging, sickness, and death. He would point out that daily life is full of aging and death: "Start allowing that in, start understanding that it is normal and natural and that you've got to come to peace with it." He got me to look at how resistant I was to doing that. I don't know if anyone's an expert on death; I'm not, but I sincerely worked on my fear of it, trying to understand it. It was very, very helpful. For me the question is always "Can you be awake to what it is that's happening to you right now?"

Q. *Who are the teachers who have been most influential in your practice?*

A. My starting point in practice was a very intellectual one. I had read a lot of books but I hadn't done any serious meditation yet. I was with my first Buddhist teacher, a Korean Zen master named Sung Zhan, who was accompanying me to Korea, where I was going to spend a year in a monastery.

On the plane I opened up my bag and picked out a book I was starting to read. He asked, "What's all that?" I said, "I have these great dharma books and I'm going to take these with me." He said, "Oh no, you *merely* understand everything already." Then he continued in his broken English, "This year, whole year, no reading." For a New York Jewish intellectual, that's like telling a junkie to go cold turkey.

Believe it or not I did it. The first few weeks were torture. I was reading ketchup bottles — "tomatoes, citric acid . . . " — just to be able to read something. Then it passed and I didn't read for the whole year. I came back and of course I'm reading again, but it's very, very different. The time away helped me clarify my understanding.

So many other teachers have had an important impact on my life and my practice. One was Krishnamurti, whom I met when he was visiting Brandeis. I was struck by his suggestion that taking care of the body was a necessary part of spiritual practice. He did yoga every day, he had a careful diet, and of course his emphasis was on awareness, very similar to Buddhist Vipassana emphasis without the methods and techniques.

The next person I met was a yogi named Badarayana. I

wanted to study the *Bhagavad-Gita* with him. He said, "Before we do that, we've got to clean you out and do some purification." He put me on a twenty-two-day fast, and coming out of it he made all kinds of suggestions about diet. He encouraged me to practice the asanas with breathing. He emphasized that the care of the physical body is not antagonistic to spiritual life, although it easily can become such if you use it for vanity. Buddhism is good because it gets you to face the body's impermanent nature, but sometimes the Buddhist side seems to regard health as incidental.

Since then, doing asanas and keeping a reasonable diet, I experience those practices as connected with my intensive meditation practice. I used to get teased, but things have changed: The Buddhists and the yogis are starting to work together, to learn from each other. I've come out of the closet as someone who has a foot in both camps.

Q. *What is the most inspiring edge of your practice these days, Larry?*

A. What inspires me most is awareness itself. It seems to me the whole path is about attention, and the willingness to learn from what you see and hear both internally and externally. I teach in Buddhist settings ninety-nine percent of the time, but it's really about an approach to living, not affiliation.

A few years ago at the end of a dharma talk someone asked me a startling question: "Are you a Buddhist?" It was this big hall full of people and I got very quiet. Then I gave the most honest answer I know: I said no. I'm a student of the teaching of the Buddha; I'm doing the very best I can to understand it and put it into practice and share it with people. If that makes me a Buddhist, fine, but what gets me really excited is self-knowing, self-knowledge, awareness — anything that helps human beings flower, that helps them go toward sanity, toward kindness, toward wisdom in this world that has become more and more insane. The word *Buddhism* doesn't come to mind, although that has been the main vehicle for me. I just feel great when somebody starts to see the value in looking into their life.

Two teachers who helped me get here are Krishnamurti and Vimala Thakar. Both of them are nonsectarian. To me they're good role models of people who are committed to taking a look at themselves, and tirelessly encouraging the rest of us not to be afraid. They talk to our strengths, and encourage us to look at whatever is there in the moment. They teach us that we can actually expand our capacity to receive our own lives in the moment. I've had a few awakenings from doing that, a glimpse of what it's like when the mind is completely free of the past and of "me" and "mine." A lot of the people I work with are at a much earlier phase in their practice, and I do my best to convey to them that there's a treasure awaiting them if they're willing to work at it.

Q. *With the long perspective you now have on practice, what would you say that treasure is?*

A. When I first started practicing I had the frame of reference that I had in graduate school: If I practice really hard, some day I'll get enlightened. And when I do, there'll be some kind of Steven Spielberg special effect, and I'll be transformed into this incredible person with no problems. It was like "Even if I'm miserable now, I'm going to be terrific someday when I become a really great yogi."

Along the way I've been influenced by a lot of different teachings within Buddhism. One is Dogen's teaching that practice and awakening are the same thing; they are simultaneous. Or, put another way, the means is the end. The essence of the practice is the practice of liberation. When you're neither craving nor pushing something away — that's a moment of freedom. The moment when you're holding on or pushing away, you're enslaved. It's all about taking care of this moment, and in Dogen's terminology the means and the ends are the same thing. When you're as awake as you can be in this moment, the whole quality of your life is different. That's the practice. I have a hunch there's no end to the learning and the unfolding of this, and that's fine with me. The path and the goal are the same.

Q. *Larry, I've known you for a number of years now, and I sense that* Metta, *or* Lovingkindness, *practice has been somehow important to you. Can you say a few words about that?*

A. I found that what helped me most of all was not formal *Metta* practice, and I would say to this day that is true. I don't do all that much formal *Metta* practice. When I finally started to enter into prolonged periods of stillness, I wasn't cultivating being a kinder person, per se; I was just learning how to soak in that fullness. I feel that my major healing around lovingkindness had to do with learning to be in the silence. I think the main healing took place in the silence itself, but I didn't know it then. I wasn't cultivating kindness; it was just something that seemed to come out of the stillness.

Another story, if I may: I was a very gentlemanly, considerate little boy. When I was eight years old, I was leaving the apartment house where I lived in Brooklyn as an elderly woman was on her way out as well, and I held the door open for her. She looked at me and said, "Well, ain't you the little gentleman," and she started laughing. Then she told my mother and this lady and that, and before I knew it everyone was saying "Ain't you the little gentleman. Larry, open the door." I got embarrassed about being openly kind and went underground; I don't think I was unkind but I had ambivalence about expressing it, and it took me years to overcome that.

Thanks to my practice I am more like what I was as a child before the school system got hold of me. And the more I meditate, the more loving I am. I think I spent the first part of my life running away from love. Today I figure if you can open a door for someone, why not? It's become easier for me to express my love.

I grew up in a very urban, noisy Brooklyn, and have always been intrigued by silence. At first I wanted external silence, but that goal soon became internal silence. It's a vast realm. People have said space, or the ocean, is the "last frontier," but I think there's another frontier — each of us is an entire universe to be explored. Enjoying the quality of stillness and joy that comes up in practice, being with whatever is there, is just wonderful.

I would say that the greatest benefits and healing really began to happen for me when I started to be able to taste silence. That came out of contemplative life, and it's still amazing to me. Silence is highly charged with a subtle form of life. You become more loving and wiser, and I don't know how that happens.

Q. *You have a reputation, Larry, for teaching a kind of "engaged silence."*

A. I'm working on learning how to go from the serene quietude of sitting out into the street. There's an interplay between the contemplative practice of sitting at home and on personal retreats and throwing myself into action and inviting people to meet me there. I think that the possible tension between contemplation and action is a necessary element of the authentic American or Western dharma that we're trying to create, which will be meaningful for lay practitioners. Most laypeople have families and full-time jobs. We all know what can be a cliché — "Be mindful of your daily life" — but we have to learn how to use our ordinary life to turn that into an actuality.

In terms of the sitting, *anapanasati* [breath awareness] has been a central method of mine for a long time. But honestly when I sit these days, within a few moments it's not about the breath at all— it has nothing to do with the breath. The breath is useful insofar as it helps develop this quality of being awake. But awake to what? Awake to my life as it is right here, right now.

A lot of people I speak with are interested in the anxieties that are brought up by what's happening now in the world: war, SARS, unemployment, terrorism. My feeling is that if this is daily life practice, then the world is not an impediment to practice: The world *is* the practice. These are the times we live in, this is a fact. This is actually happening, what's going on right now. It's actually true, and we need to accept it. We can spend our time blaming the president, talking to the TV — I do that sometimes too — but it doesn't get us anywhere. The point is not to take a certain political view, but to stay clear so that you can live your life as best you can, including how you relate to political issues.

If we're to have a genuine lay practice, then we have to practice with what's going on, and this is what's going on. Thich Nhat Hanh talks beautifully about refugees from Vietnam, who would leave on these rickety boats. Some boats would make it and some wouldn't. What they discovered is, if there was at least one person who could remain calm during the turbulent seas, that boat had a much better chance of getting through. We're all yogis, we're all special forces. You're that one person in the boat in your world right now; but the only way you can be that person is to use this practice. I'm not advocating any political philosophy, I'm advocating that you use the practice for your own life.

There's a Hasidic teaching that might be helpful here. It is "God assigns a small sector of the universe to each one of us to take care of." You each know what your little part of the world is, so your job is to take care of that. Face what is. See exactly what's happening right now, and see what is needed. ●

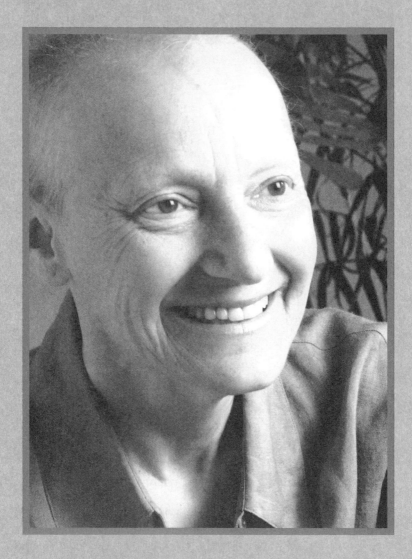

Esther Myers

COMING HOME TO MY BODY, TO MYSELF

ESTHER MYERS says that one of the blessings in her life has been meeting the right people at the right time. When she returned to Toronto in 1976 intending to teach yoga, it was a very unusual career choice. She was helped by a career counselor who encouraged her to "go for it" in the earliest days of teaching. • Lynn Wylie helped Esther start her writing career by coauthoring a practice manual for beginners, *The Ground, the Breath and the Spine,* which was self-published. It gradually evolved into *Yoga and You.* • Esther felt that her teacher Vanda Scaravelli's wave movement couldn't be adequately communicated in words. In 1993, with the help of Kim Echlin and Vanda's grandson, David Cohen, Esther produced a documentary video about Vanda. • Esther's latest inspiration came from two friends from very different parts of her life who asked what her practice was like after her mastectomy. The answer is unprintable. They both advised her to write from that place. The result was an article in *Yoga Journal* in December 1998. Recently she produced a video titled *Gentle Yoga for Breast Cancer Survivors.* Esther is author of *Hands-On Manual for Teachers* and is now working on a book that explores more fully her experience and the evolution of her practice.

THIRTY YEARS OF PRACTICE have taught me that yoga offers no guarantees. It has not guaranteed me health, a beautiful body, or longevity.

In 1994 I was diagnosed with breast cancer and had a mastectomy along with the removal of some lymph nodes from my right armpit. That was followed by a hysterectomy in 1999 for removal of an ovarian tumor. In March of 2001, I was diagnosed with spread of the breast cancer into my abdominal and pleural cavities. The tumor in my abdomen is sizable and both tumors have adhesions, which have restricted my movement and breathing. As I write this in March 2003, I am undergoing chemotherapy.

When I was first diagnosed with cancer, I was shocked. I felt that I had been doing everything right: I had a good diet, practiced yoga, had a healthy lifestyle, and held a relatively stress-free job. That's when I learned that yoga offers no guarantees.

I was first drawn to yoga as a means of helping me sit comfortably on the floor. In January 1972 I was twenty-five and living in London, England. I moved into the Archway community, one of a number of intentional communities, developed under the auspices of Dr. R. D. Laing, a radical psychiatrist who envisioned the communities as true asylums — places where one could retreat for protection and healing.

I was attracted to this community because of the willingness of its members to strip away roles, norms, and conventions in order to find the truth at the heart of their experience. I had no idea until many years later that that is also the goal of yoga and meditation.

As part of the hippie aspect of the community, people sat on the floor for meals, meetings, and seminars. I was surprised that so many people found it comfortable. I didn't. When Arthur Balaskas offered us a free yoga class, I decided to take it, thinking that it would help me sit on the floor more easily. I was right.

The classes were in Iyengar yoga, now known for its precision and attention to details of structure and alignment. I learned the poses quickly and easily. I loved its dynamic energy. I took to its relentless challenge to extend and improve like a duck to water.

Looking back now, I am struck by the immediate resonance I had with the archetypal forms of the postures. Although I didn't realize it at the time, I had found my way, and discovered a practice that gave, and continues to give, focus, meaning, direction, and purpose to my life.

In 1974 I began studying with Mary Stewart, author of *Yoga for Children* and *Yoga Over 50,* and did most of my training in Iyengar yoga with her in London. When I completed my training in 1976, I returned to my native Toronto and began to teach. I was one of the first Iyengar teachers in Toronto, and found myself instantly teaching teachers who were also drawn to the precision and challenge of the Iyengar Method. I returned to Europe annually for continued lessons.

In 1978 I was introduced to Vanda Scaravelli, author of *Awakening the Spine,* at her home just outside Fiesole in the hills overlooking Florence, Italy. Vanda had studied with B. K. S. Iyengar and T. K. V. Desikachar in the early 1960s, then set out to find her own way: a yoga that is simultaneously gentle and dynamic.

Using the breath as her guide, Vanda discovered a movement within the postures that integrated the flow of breath and the curving of the spine to create a powerful undulation through the poses.

In 1984 she came to Toronto to visit her daughter and I had my first lessons with her. For the next ten years, she came to Toronto annually in the summer and stayed for three or four months. I had lessons with her three times a week while she was here.

Vanda taught as she had learned from Mr. Iyengar: one-to-one, body-to-body. Studying with her demanded a level of trust and surrender that I had never experienced before. Vanda was an extraordinary role model in following her passion, trusting her process, and accessing the extraordinary possibilities of the human body, regardless of age. She showed me dynamic and expressive potential in asana practice that I had never seen or imagined.

> "Although I didn't realize it at the time, I had found my way, and discovered a practice that gave, and continues to give, focus, meaning, direction, and purpose to my life."

She was seventy-eight when I began studying with her, and transmitting her discovery before she died was a core issue in her life. I took on the mantle readily.

My first challenge was to integrate her approach into my practice and later to translate what I had learned into a class or workshop setting. The deeper challenges came when my annual lessons stopped and I was working on my own without a teacher. I began to acknowledge my profound sense of emptiness, and the feeling that I could not begin to access the powerful energy she had tapped into. Very slowly that has changed.

"Yoga has not offered me any quick fixes or easy solutions."

Vanda did not want her work named. She said that she had studied with Mr. Iyengar and then found her own way. She told me that I should take her work and find my own way. That brought my inner critic to the fore. I found myself confronting a relentless voice that asked: "Who do you think you are?"

The diagnosis of cancer and subsequent mastectomy in the spring of 1994 brought new challenges to my yoga practice. The first was deciding on what kind of treatment to have. My surgeon said I could take my time making a decision. Even in the midst of my terror and confusion, I knew that I could reach a clear, quiet place in which I would know what to do, and that I should wait until that happened.

The mastectomy changed my body overnight. I was suddenly exhausted and barely able to move my right arm. I was used to a strong practice and had no resources for dealing with my new state. The surgery forced me to learn to listen to my body and respect its limitations. This lesson was repeated after the hysterectomy and again with the spread of the disease. Before I started chemotherapy, my breathing was becoming increasingly restricted. I was no longer practicing to do the poses; I was practicing in order to breathe.

The combination of losing a breast, my ovaries, and uterus and the physical changes of menopause made me realize how deeply I was identified with the Western ideal of an attractive body. Furthermore, the undulating movement that Vanda incorporated in the postures was fluid, organic, and quintessentially feminine. I questioned what it meant to be a woman and the relationship of my sexuality to my yoga practice.

In the last nine years I have gone through long periods where my practice consisted primarily of passive and restful poses, and relaxation. Another golden opportunity for my inner critic. I so often feel that I should be practicing longer, or more deeply, or doing more advanced practices.

At the moment I average an hour to an hour and a half a day of practice, including about half an hour of sitting. My practice is very gradual. If I overdo it, especially with back bends, my abdomen recoils in spasm.

The last nine years have brought me face-to-face with so many physical and emotional challenges. My practice has highlighted my deepest fears and insecurities; it is often hard to get back on the mat. I have yearned for the innocent joy I felt in my practice when I began over thirty years ago.

Yoga has not offered me any quick fixes or easy solutions. One of my students asked me recently if my yoga practice has been sufficient to sustain me through these health crises. The answer: Absolutely not. In addition to extraordinary support from students, colleagues, family, and friends, I have made extensive use of conventional medicine, naturopathic medicine, traditional Chinese medicine, psychotherapy, bodywork, and other healing modalities.

Very gradually I have found moments of being at peace with the limitations in my movement and energy, and a deeper appreciation of the richness of my life. At Kripalu's 2002 Yoga and Buddhism Conference, Buddhist teacher Robert Hall spoke of learning to live a happy life while looking death in the eye. I thought, "Yes."

Finding ways to alleviate my own suffering, become more truly myself, and help others find their way is a key goal of my practice and teaching. On a global level, it's hard to imagine how I can make a difference. When I think about the violence and suffering in the world, as well as the state of the environment, I find it difficult not to sink into despair and helplessness.

On a personal level, however, I have seen changes in my students that are gratifying and often humbling. Many of my students have left more conventional or lucrative jobs to become yoga teachers. Others have made major life changes that have helped them live more authentic and satisfying lives. One of my students came out as a lesbian as a result of her yoga practice.

Another student told me recently about a class she was teaching for people with post-polio syndrome. One day one of the students unexpectedly brought her husband, who is paraplegic, to class. As my student scrambled to figure out what she could teach that would include him, she thought: "Yoga is love. How can I love him?" She decided to teach alternate nostril breathing, since he has the use of one arm. After the class he told her that before his accident he had been a diver. Breathing was a practice he understood deeply.

As I listened to her story, I felt that I was in the presence of an extraordinary teacher. I wondered, "Who is the teacher here and who is the student?" To my amazement, upon completing her story, she turned to me and said: "Esther, I learned that from you." ●

"Finding ways to alleviate
my own suffering, become more truly
myself, and help others find
their way is a key goal
of my practice and teaching."

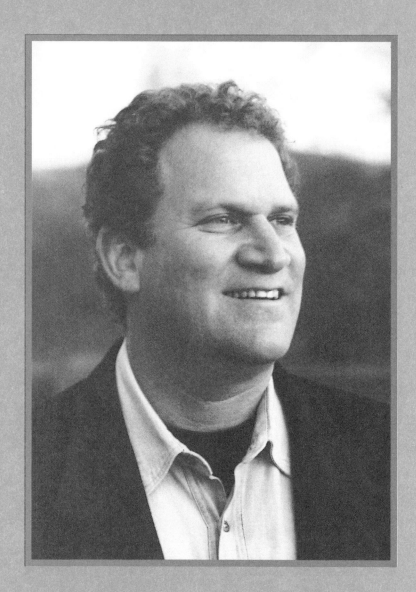

Lama Surya Das

CHANGING EVERYTHING; CHANGING NOTHING

LAMA SURYA DAS is one of the foremost Western Buddhist meditation teachers and scholars. Born Jeffrey Miller, he was raised in Valley Stream on New York's Long Island, where he celebrated his bar mitzvah and earned letters in basketball, baseball, and soccer at Valley Stream Central High School (class of 1968). While a student at the State University of New York at Buffalo, he attended antiwar protests, marched on Washington, and attended Woodstock. After graduating with honors from college, he traveled throughout Europe and the East, and he has spent nearly thirty years studying Zen, Vipassana, yoga, and Tibetan Buddhism with many of the great old masters of Asia. • Today, Lama Surya Das teaches and lectures around the world. Based on his relationship with His Holiness the Dalai Lama, Surya Das founded the Western Buddhist Teachers Network and has organized three week-long conferences of Western Buddhist Meditation Teachers with the Dalai Lama in Dharamsala, India. • Surya Das is the author of *Awakening the Buddha Within: Eight Steps to Enlightenment, Awakening to the Sacred: Building a Spiritual Life from Scratch,* and *Awakening the Buddhist Heart: Integrating Love, Meaning, and Connection into Every Part of Your Life.* • He lives in Arlington, Massachusetts.

PEOPLE SOMETIMES ASK ME what difference practice has made in my life. The answer is it's changed everything for me. And, in a funny way, it's changed nothing.

Here's a story: On his deathbed, my late guru, the Sixteenth Karmapa, the Grand Lama who was head of the Kagyu sect of Tibetan Buddhism, said to his disciples, "Nothing happens." What was the unspoken question that the disciple in front of him was asking with his eyes that brought forth that answer? Was it: "What happens when the Master dies?" "What happens at death?" "What happens in the mystery of life in this universe?" The words the Master spoke were: "Nothing happens." And that sort of sums it all up: Nothing happens and yet it's all going on.

I learned to meditate at college in the late '60s, but I couldn't really follow through with it as a daily practice. In 1971 I started Vipassana meditation retreats with S. N. Goenka in India and vowed to meditate every day. Making that vow and doing it every day since then has totally changed my life. That's the good news.

The bad news, if you want to put it that way, is that really nothing changes. In the early '70s I came back from my first three-year stint in India and I was all full of myself. My younger brother, the scientist, said, "Surya, you're still yourself." I felt deflated; my shoulders drooped. Then he said, ". . . but even more so." So that was the good news as well as the bad news.

I've come to trust, to believe with conviction, that nothing fundamentally affects my true nature. That's the good news the Dharma has brought me that's changed everything. As a result, things come and go and flow more peaceably, and I'm more at ease with them — at harmony and at peace. That's been the greatest satisfaction in my life.

So in one way practice has changed my life and in another way it has taught me that there is no other life. I give all praise to the dharma. I'm not talking about Buddhism or Hinduism, or any other "-ism," or the religions built around those thoughts, but rather the practice — the daily and other practices that have changed my life.

The source of my deepest inspiration is my root guru. Most of my gurus are gone now, although some are purportedly reborn. I also draw inspiration from my late Dzogchen Master, Nyoshul Khenpo Rinpoche, who passed away two and a half years ago at our retreat center in Southern France. He's very alive for me.

All my gurus are very much with me — they never really died. The bodies died but the guru principle lives, and that's very important; that's very close to me, very inspiring and motivating. Especially in these benighted times in our fast-paced, postmodern society, being connected to that timeless principle makes all the difference to me.

Spiritual community is important for us as well today, especially since most Westerners are non-monastic, not hermits. Spiritual community and, by extension, spiritual family can be very important. Being part of a community helps keep our hearts open. We need our practice communities, of course, but I think we need to create community beyond those little enclaves. We need to work for, aspire toward, and connect our hands and heads and hearts in creating spiritual community in a larger sense.

Lately I'm seeing much more activism, much more emphasis

on "how do we transform the world and not just our own little enclave." I'm heartened by that. It's important. Of course the shadow side of that is that we get even busier. I hate to see engaged Buddhists being like enraged Buddhists — fighting and kicking ass for peace. It seems a contradiction in terms.

If we can tame our nature, gentle our nature, and disarm our hearts, then we really can be peaceful spiritual activists and enlightened leaders. I'm all for that. I think we need to be cultivating enlightened leaders and fellowship, not just followers, if we want a better future. I'm all for activism and *seva,* as we call it in Sanskrit: selfless service and serving God through serving humanity and the environment and all creatures.

> "In one way practice has changed my life and in another way it has taught me that there is no other life."

I want to emphasize that for me it is very important to maintain a daily practice. I have to come from a deep connected core, a core of spiritual practice. That's why I always bring it back to daily practice — and annual or seasonal retreats. Study and practice together keep the connection deep. Otherwise we get wider and broader but it gets a little thinned out.

I meditate every morning. I do Dzogchen meditation. It's a little bit of chanting and some breathing and sometimes some yoga.

I did a two-week retreat at my hermitage in Texas this winter. I did yoga every morning, a lot of meditation, some Tibetan chanting, and a little bit of visualization. Mostly it is pure awareness practice, without form or ritual.

I think that a truly transformative spirituality today has to be very personal and not just a matter of joining a club or being a member of a movement or following the latest fads.

One way to make practice personal is to discover what way of meditation, what practice, is most "natural" for us. Some people might say, "I can't meditate, I can't sit still." But they love to sit and look at a lake, at the stars, at their sleeping child. So there's a way of being totally present that comes naturally to many people. Some people prefer yoga or Tai Chi meditation. It may be sacred music or dance; it may be connecting with nature.

All of those are natural awareness and centering and "presencing" practices. That is the way we can find our personal and authentic spirituality: using what I call natural meditations. You don't have to close your eyes or cross your legs in order to experience that.

This kind of experience is possible for everybody. Everybody is a living spirit. Everybody has a natural dharma or yoga, if they can just find it. Just as everybody has a vocation, even though many feel that they're still looking for it, so everybody has or could have a spiritual calling, a sacred path that they can find.

I've noticed that all of a sudden the whole country is chanting. That's a great practice, too. In a way it's better for most Americans than meditation; I go with my wife and we sit for three hours chanting and moving. It's almost un-American to sit still and quiet. But chanting-yoga has really come on strong, maybe because it's a natural practice for a lot of people. These are things we need to find out: ways of practice that are authentically ourselves and that we can really do.

The best practices are the ones that we do and that do us. If we can't do them, there's no point in talking about what's the best practice, the highest practice, the deepest practice — it's nonsense. What matters is what we can really do.

Over the years, meditation, yoga, chant, and prayer have helped me to calm, clear, and free my mind; purify, harmonize, and sometimes even heal my body; open my heart; and awaken my energy. They have gradually transformed my whole way of seeing and being. The balance, concentration, self-awareness, and wisdom gained through meditation practice have brought me everything I was looking for in this life, and have helped me to fulfill my purpose and reason for being in this world. I don't leave home without them!

So when my late guru said, "Nothing happens," that was kind of a koan, a nondual statement. You can cogitate on it from every angle, endlessly, and go beyond the mind that way.

That's the meaning of great emptiness, or *shunyata,* in Buddhism. Of course everything's going on — it's dreamlike, it's illusory; we can't really say for sure what it is or isn't — but at the base nothing happens. Nothing happens, but it sure is something, ain't it? ●

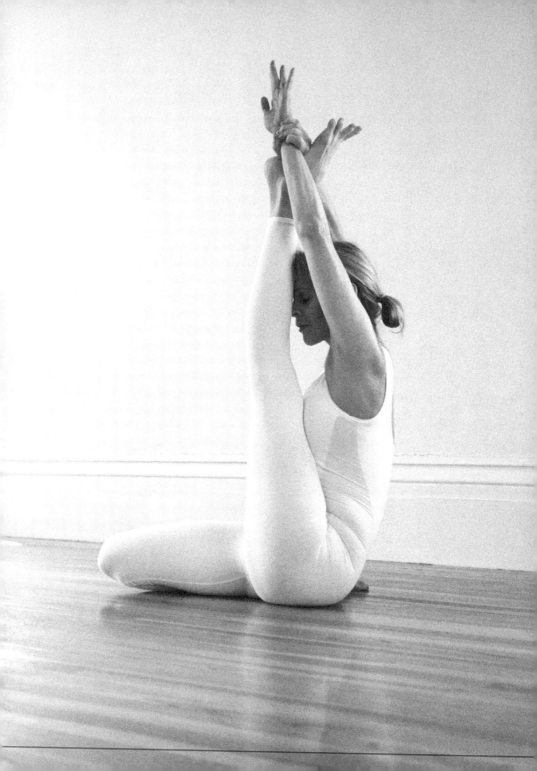

Patricia Walden

MOVING FROM DARKNESS INTO LIGHT

PATRICIA WALDEN is one of the most senior teachers in the Iyengar yoga method and is renowned for her international retreats, teacher trainings, and workshops. As one of only two Americans to hold a senior advanced teaching certificate in her tradition, she continues to have a close relationship with her teacher, Yogacharya B. K. S. Iyengar. • Patricia was born in Newton, Massachusetts. She graduated in the early '70s from the streets of San Francisco, where she had been a student of Murshid Sam Lewis ("Sufi Sam"). In 1976 she met Yogacharya B. K. S. Iyengar and immersed herself in practice. Since then, she has studied with him almost annually in India, and has also studied intensively with Dona Holleman in Florence, Italy. • Along with her teaching, Patricia is known for her yoga videos, including *Yoga for Beginners*, and for her writings, including *Women's Book of Yoga and Health* (with Linda Sparrowe). She was cited by *Yoga Journal* as one of the "Twenty-five American Yoga Originals who are shaping yoga today," and was featured in *Time* magazine for her work with yoga and healing. Patricia has a special interest in yoga for women and yoga for depression. • She currently lives with her partner, Tom Alden, in a two-story brick cave in Cambridge with their one Ganesh and three Quan Yins.

Q. *How has practice changed your life, Patricia?*

A. I would have to say that yoga has changed my life dramatically. And that's not an exaggeration. When I was in my twenties I was in therapy for depression. I remember the therapist telling me probably two years into my therapy with him that my depression was hereditary, and that I would probably always have it. I got really angry. That comment made me feel as though I had a label on my T-shirt that said DEPRESSION FOREVER. In the last ten years, though, that visitor — depression — has not come to me again. I no longer suffer from depression, and it's definitely because of my yoga practice.

This is astonishing to me, especially when I think of where I was as a child, and in my teens and twenties. In those years there was definitely more darkness than light. I feel very blessed and very grateful to have come through it. It hasn't been easy. In fact it's been hard work. And by the way, just because you have a spiritual discipline doesn't mean that you will necessarily be transformed. One has to be willing to practice and to look at oneself deeply and clearly.

One of the biggest changes in my life is that I can live with impermanence now. I don't always have to know the outcome in order to feel safe. I am much more adaptable. I can live with not knowing, and know deep in my heart that whatever happens I am going to be OK. It think this comes from having faith in God, faith in the universe, that no matter what happens I am going to be supported and I am going to be OK.

I think that developing this deep sense of OK-ness is particularly difficult for people who grow up in dysfunctional homes or in homes where there's alcoholism. For children growing up in those environments, any change can bring on incredible anxiety. When I was in my teens and twenties, any change could push me over an edge. If I was in a place of not knowing, that always scared me.

About sixteen years ago, though, I consciously began to take more risks in my life. At the time there was still fear; now the fear is much less. For example, right now I'm in the process of giving up my yoga center, which has been my world and my life. It is a risk, and I'm fine with it and open to the future. That's one of my mantras: "supported by the past, seated in the present, and open to whatever the future has for me."

Q. *Some say that when you grow up in a traumatic situation, there's a certain brain chemistry that is imprinted at a very young age. Do you believe that yoga actually changes that?*

A. Yes. In the last few years I've been doing depression workshops around the country, and that's one of the things that I work with: how what we do with our bodies can change our brain chemistry. Candace Pert, author of *Molecules of Emotion,* has studied how thinking affects feeling and how physiology affects thinking. I have had direct experience with that. If I'm low in energy or feeling melancholy, I do back bends. When I'm finished I feel wonderful. Or, if I feel scattered and agitated, I do forward bends and I feel rebalanced.

Doing these postures repeatedly changes your brain chemistry over time. Just a simple thing such as keeping your chest lifted and not frowning has been shown to affect your brain chemistry.

One of the things yoga teaches us is that how our body is now is a direct result of experiences we've had in the past. It works the other way around as well. What we're doing with our body now will determine our body in the future. Every feeling, every thought, every action that we take is deepening a groove; whether it's a positive feeling or a negative feeling, the groove gets deeper.

Q. *Have you always been aware that moving your physical body could affect your thinking and feelings?*

A. I did have a difficult childhood. On the one hand I was very timid, but on the other hand I was very powerful and strong. I learned how to dance when I was around nine years old and I realized that when I danced, I felt joyful. This was just freestyle dance with my friends. We'd imitate things we saw in movies or just play around or dance to records. When I danced I got out of myself. I had so much fun and thought, "This is actually a way for me not to feel bad." It was like getting out of myself into my body, and into the joy of living.

Now, at fifty-six, I use the same vehicle — my body, my instrument — to go deeper into myself. As a young person I used dance and movement to get away; now I use it to move toward myself — I might even say, toward the Self. I'm still using my body to feel better, but the approach is different.

Q. *How did you make the shift from dance into yoga?*

A. To be perfectly honest, I loved dance, but I wasn't really that great at it, and I didn't feel fully satisfied with it. I was always wanting more when I was dancing, and that's actually when I became more serious about it. But after I started taking it seriously it wasn't so much fun anymore.

During the time I was dancing, I took my first yoga class. Shoulder Stand was one of the first poses taught and I remember feeling a fullness in that pose that's hard to put into words — just a feeling of complete satisfaction and surrender and warmth. I felt very nurtured. When I found out years later that Shoulder Stand is called "the mother of the asanas, the yoga postures" it was very interesting to me because that's how I felt: mothered. I felt absolutely full and OK. It also felt familiar, like "Oh, I've done this before."

That was the beginning of my experience of yoga. What I felt in an asana that was different from dance was that in dance I felt great but I didn't have an internal connection, while in the asana I felt wonderful in my body but I also felt my existence from the inside. Through asanas I began to be able to look into myself and feel OK with it.

Q. *So somehow the yoga mat became a safe space for you.*

A. Absolutely. I can't tell you the number of times in my twenties when I was in one crisis or another and I'd go to my mat and it always soothed me. I usually did Shoulder Stand when I was in crisis. When I did that pose, I felt "Things are going to be OK. You're going to be OK."

Q. *Why was the soothing aspect so important to you?*

A. Many children of alcoholics don't feel OK and don't feel soothed. That's what we're either consciously or unconsciously looking for. In my early twenties I did hard drugs. I did heroin and it wasn't to party: I was essentially self-medicating. Then I learned that asanas can do that as well. It's a slower process — the holistic path is always slower — but of course it's much better. Heroin just unplugs you and you don't feel anything, but when you do a series of yoga asanas, you feel good, you feel soothed—and you really are soothed physiologically.

Q. *Did this soothing experience lead you deeper into your yoga practice?*

A. Yes. It is still a form of self-soothing, but it has become much more than that for me. Not that I never need to be soothed these days; I do, of course. But I feel better now in my life, so my yoga practice takes me deeper than that.

In my early twenties when I first started teaching yoga, I wasn't leading a so-called yoga lifestyle, although I was practicing occasionally and teaching. I was actually leading two lives. I was still doing drugs intermittently. I was still feeling depressed. I was not caring for myself in good ways, although I was trying to. I had my life of going to teach my classes and practicing, but I had another dark life and a dark mind. There was a big gap between my inner life and my outer life, so I felt like a fake much of the time. It is agonizing when you're going to a class and teaching yoga and you know you're not living it a hundred percent, even though you really believe in it.

One of the biggest things that happened to me in my midtwenties was that I slowly began to practice more and get out of the dark world I was in. Slowly, slowly, slowly my inner life and my outer life were mirroring each other. Now the person I am out there in the world is the same person I am when I'm teaching and when I'm home by myself. They are all connected.

Q. *What I hear in your story is a kind of gradual attunement to your own naturally arising impulses and needs and internal life.*

A. I think that most kids who grow up in dysfunctional families like mine feel very alone. You have to figure things out for yourself: how to nurture yourself, how to take care of yourself. It has some benefits, of course. As a result of my experience, I'm a survivor. I'm very strong willed. I have always been strong willed, and I was very angry when I was in my twenties.

Anger is just another form of energy. Through my practice of yoga — and through my relationship with Murshid Sam Lewis and my Sufi training — I was able to channel this powerful force, this energy inside me, and direct it toward something positive. Anger is such a powerful energy that if you can channel it toward something positive, it's remarkable. And there's a lot of clarity in anger. I really think that at my angriest I have also often been at my clearest!

Q. *How have the traditions of yoga helped you make this transition?*

A. The teachings and some of the ancient scriptures helped me a lot — especially the *Upanishads.* There is a wonderful new commentary called *Katha Upanishad* by Swami Ambikananda Saraswati. She talks about the path in the shade and the path in the light. The path in the shade is when you're looking outside yourself to find happiness or to be soothed or whatever. The path in the light is when you realize buying clothes or doing drugs or whatever brings you momentary pleasure, but is not really the way. It may feel wonderful momentarily, but once you have spent five- hundred dollars on a cashmere sweater and you've worn it five times, then it's only a matter of time until you want the next one — and the next. It's nice to have those things, but they're not going to bring you lasting happiness or fulfillment. When I look deep inside and practice even when I don't want to, I connect with the fullness, peace, and love that is our true nature.

Many years ago, when I was fifty percent in the drug world and fifty percent in the yoga world, I had some of my darkest moments. Even then I was learning to pause and say, "OK, if I do this drug, how am I going to feel a week from now? On the other hand, if I go to my mat and do Headstand, how am I going to feel a week from now?" The ability to step back, to look at your life, to pause and do that little bit of meditation, and then make your choice according to how you want your future to be is one of the things I learned early on. It is so powerful, that little moment of freedom and grace where for whatever reason you are able to pause before making your decision. Then, of course, as we mature on the path our choices are different.

Today my choices are no longer "Am I going to do heroin or am I going to practice?" They're different kinds of choices. Now I ask myself, "OK, what is going to bring me closer to myself, or to enlightenment?" That was the kind of inquiry that helped me decide whether or not to continue with my yoga center. One of the things I want to do in my life is to grow spiritually, to be kinder, to be more compassionate, and to have my life set up in such a way that I have a better chance of cultivating those qualities. I am fortunate to have choices. And I know that giving up the center has been just the right thing for me. It was wonderful for many years but now I'm entering a new chapter in my life.

Q. *How did you learn to trust your inner feelings?*

A. It's been a long, powerful, painful, and wonderful journey. It's taken years to be able to trust my own voice and not look to other people to tell me how to feel or how to act or what to do. It's the time I've spent on my mat practicing — even when I didn't feel like it — and also my relationship with my teacher B. K. S. Iyengar that has helped me. He challenged me to go deeper into myself.

There's something about his energy and our relationship that helped me face my own demons and my own karma. I will be forever grateful to him for that. One of his most important mantras — one that he used a lot in his early days of teaching — was "Take an action. No matter how small, just take one action."

Q. *Clearly you allowed yourself to enter into a profound teacher/student relationship with Mr. Iyengar and it transformed you.*

A. It really did, and it continues to. It's interesting because he is a fierce teacher. He is also a compassionate teacher. He has very high standards. I met him in my twenties when I was not in a good place. I presented myself as being all together and he saw very soon that I was a fragile and weak person. There is something about his fire that brought out my own. His fire ignited my fire and gave me strength.

Q. *You saw something in him that you knew was also in yourself?*

A. That's exactly right. I think I saw fully developed in him something that I knew was also in me, but in seed form. I think that's what good teachers do. They are able to bring the strong qualities, those wonderful qualities, out of their students. Sometimes we find those qualities through imitating our teachers. Sometimes it's the teacher's words or example. But that's clearly what Mr. Iyengar did for me.

Q. *You're still very much in relationship with him?*

A. Yes. I see him every year and our relationship is a wonderful one. It's clear that he loves me. I feel it in his presence, and he's proud of all the work I've done. He ignored me for the first five or six years that I went to India. That was so painful for me because I loved him so much. I decided that no matter what, I was going to make him see me and notice me. That was part of my impetus to practice. That is part of how I became a strong practitioner.

I feel truly blessed to have taken my journey with Mr. Iyengar. From the very beginning until now, to have a teacher who was seeing me at my worst, watching me grow, acknowledging that I was growing and that "Oh you could take this next step," "What you're doing is really good," "You've changed, but now go there, now go here," and "Don't just keep it physical," that "This is just your instrument. You're on a precipice now," "Now go a little bit deeper inside." It's been wonderful.

He's eighty-four now, and his practice has been very strong up until this last year. When I go to Puna, I go primarily to practice near him or with him. I always put myself right beside him at the institute. Sometimes I follow along with him and sometimes I don't, but he'll always come and adjust me and take me to the next step.

Last December, when I went to say good-bye to him (He always hits me on the head. It feels like shakti. Then he laughs this childlike laugh), he said to me, "Well, who's going to inspire me to practice now?" I fell to my knees weeping because it had come full circle. Of course he said it in a joking way. It was a compliment to me, though. I think he meant "Oh, you've worked really hard and what you're doing is good."

Q. *You're mirrors for each other. He clearly saw something in you just as you saw something in him.*

A. When I'm in his presence, he doesn't have to say anything. He can be luminous and I feel when I'm in his light that I become light as well, and even more so when he's practicing. I recently realized I'm not only attached to him as my teacher and inspiration and as a human being, but I'm attached to his practice. That has given me a fire to go on. I do have my own fire but I realize that when he's no longer practicing and I can no longer sit beside him and watch him practice, that is going to be a major loss. So I'm working to let go of that for myself, but also for him. As people age, we have to let them age and not pull on them or hold too tightly.

I also feel with Guruji that I am part of a lineage and I love that. I honor that lineage, and he is giving more and more responsibility to me. It's very interesting and a little bit daunting when the roles change, when your teacher is passing you the torch. For years I've leaned on my teacher and looked to him for guidance and inspiration, but now he's saying "No. Now you have to take this and bring it out to your students. You can't rely on me anymore."

Part of me wants to keep my relationship with him the same, but isn't this change a part of life? Relationships change. When you're in the midst of it there is some discomfort and some effort to find your own way and your own voice within it. That's where I am right now in our relationship. I'd like to share a few lines of a Rumi poem, called "You Are Not a Single You."

> This world is a tree and we are green, half-ripe
>   fruit on it.
>
> We hold tight to the limbs because we know we
>   are not ready to be taken into the palace.
>
> When we mature and sweeten we'll feel
>   ashamed to having clung so clingingly.
>
> To hold fast is a sure sign of unripeness.
>
> To drink and enjoy blood is fine for an embryo.

When I was reading this poem, I was thinking of myself as a young girl and young woman. I was reminded that even in my twenties when I'd go to my parents' house and sit at the dinner table or sit around having conversation, my fingers were always drawn in to my palms, sort of like a clenched fist. I realized that I was trying to hold on in their presence. And I took that out into my life. My hands were almost always clenched because I was holding on, trying to keep it all together. I realize now that I'm not clenching my palms anymore. My palms are relaxed.

Q. *What do you see as the growing edge of your practice right now?*

A. I have a teacher-training program and for the last six months we've been working with one of the *niyamas,* the internal restraints that are the second limb of Patanjali's Eight Limbs of Yoga. The particular *niyama* we're practicing is *ishvara pranidhana,* which is translated "Surrender to God." I've been exploring that in my asana practice, my *pranayama* practice, and also meditation, asking myself, as I've done for probably thirty-five years of my life, "What is God to me?"

I have realized that I find God when I'm doing *pranayama* practice or meditation. Grace flows spontaneously then. I'm able to go underneath my feelings and my thoughts, and experience this deep, deep feeling of spaciousness and silence. It doesn't happen all the time, but it happens more and more that I'm able to rest in this spaciousness and this profound silence. I think the keys for me are spaciousness, lightness, and silence. I equate spaciousness and silence with experiencing divine presence.

That's where I am right now. These days, actually, I don't think of my practice in terms of where I am going with it. It's more about where it is going with me! But I'm glad to say that right now I am in a wonderful and fresh new place with it. Practice is always new. ●

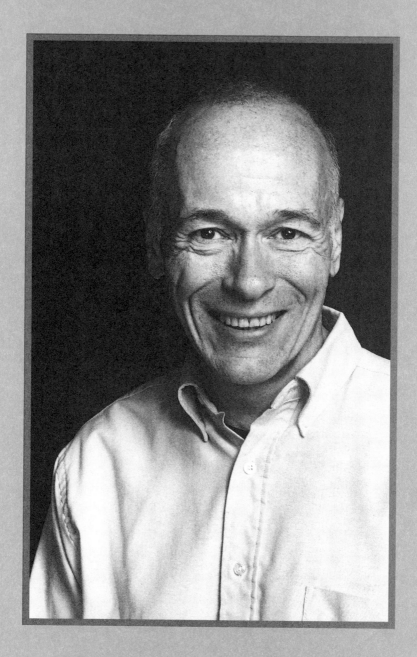

Douglas Phillips

THE TRUTH-TELLING PLACE OF EVERYDAY LIFE

DOUGLAS PHILLIPS is a clinical psychologist and a teacher of the Anapanasati approach to meditation in the Vipassana tradition. Born in Columbus, Indiana, he fell in love with Asian martial arts and culture at the age of eighteen with his introduction to competitive judo and subsequent training for twenty-five years in Chinese martial arts and non-violent self-defense. In 1975 this interest took him to Taiwan for an intensive two-year study of martial arts as well as Buddhist and Taoist meditation practices. • A growing interest in meditation and contemplative prayer led Doug to graduate degrees in comparative religious studies, divinity, ordination as an Episcopal priest, and eventually to his first Zen teacher, Maurine Stuart. Upon her death in 1990, he began study with George Bowman, with whom he took Jukai (or lay ordination), and Larry Rosenberg. His continuing association with Larry led to a deep love of Vipassana, the teachings of J. Krishnamurti, the practice of Viniyoga, and eventual training in and permission to teach Vipassana. • Doug now divides his time between teaching small groups and retreats in the New England area and a private psychotherapy practice in Newton, Massachusetts. He has been married for thirty-four years and has two adult daughters, Jessica and Megan.

LIKE MANY DRAWN TO SPIRITUAL PRACTICE, I came looking for something that would help me cope more effectively with fear, anger, insecurity, and a sense of self-in-relationship that felt deeply unsatisfying. Partly because of an early interest in martial arts and all things Asian, I was first attracted to Zen Buddhism, which became an enduring love. I imagined that by doing the practices, wearing the clothes, and chanting the chants, there would be a transformation that would liberate me from the confines of my limited and painful life experiences.

It took many years to realize that despite "experiences" of realization, my central problems were rooted in a deep sense of inadequacy, fed by fear and self-loathing, which would not be ameliorated by any outward form or "accomplishments." They would not even be changed by "realization," which meant to me at the time certain experiences that fit the descriptions I had read in the literature and heard about from fellow practitioners.

Indeed what was most liberating during this period — as I struggled with sleepiness and agitation on the cushion, and a growing family, my work, and graduate school off the cushion — was a traditional psychoanalysis of four and a half years. This analysis gave me the structure and support to face, work through, and put into perspective the painful emotional injuries and scars from childhood and adolescence, which knowingly and unknowingly undercut most of what I was trying to accomplish in day-to-day living. Psychoanalysis was my first powerful experience of genuine liberation, and without it I doubt that my life would have unfolded in the ways that have been so interesting and satisfying — including deepening access to the wisdom traditions of Zen and Vipassana, or insight meditation. This, however, does not tell the whole tale.

After analysis and completion of my doctorate, the death of my Zen teacher led me to seek another teacher, and I came to Vipassana practice. Luckily for me this new teacher had a commitment to the actualization of practice in daily living. He believed that genuine practice was possible for a layperson living in and deeply committed to a family as well as that lay practice. He believed that lay practice had to be actualized where one was *actually living.*

I found this an interesting and challenging contrast to many teachers who directly or indirectly seemed to suggest that family life was really a hindrance, and that "real" practice that was sufficiently intensive to develop deep understanding and awakening could realistically only take place in retreat and monastic settings and with regular practice in a *sangha.* The pressure in those settings was toward lots of *sesshin* and long residential retreats. This was not terribly encouraging for someone with a job, wife, children, bills, and all the other accoutrements of family life.

So for me practice became not only the commitment to daily sitting, mindfulness, and retreats when possible, but an ongoing inquiry into how I was actually living my life moment to moment. How did I spend my free time? How and what was I eating, drinking, and otherwise ingesting? Where were the occurrences of my emotional reactivity? How did I really relate to family, friends, other drivers on the road (still a growing edge of my practice!), the beggar in the street, and the person in the tollbooth? Precisely how was my on-the-cushion practice related to my off-the-cushion day-to-day living practice? How did the actualities of my daily living differ from my growing understanding of dharma and self? If there were differences between what I understood and how I lived, and there were and are many, what did I do about that?

This kind of inquiry was actually quite congruent with my previous Zen training in which I was constantly asked to demonstrate my understanding in seated meditation, walking, koan practice, and working in the kitchen and the garden. It was also a bit new for me: It was a truly intensive practice in which everything, every relationship, and every activity and behavior became a mirror reflecting me back to myself exactly as I was and am.

This was new! Everything and every encounter was "practice," not for some enlightenment in the future, but an opportunity and challenge to awaken to the dharma right now. Freedom did not have to wait! Dharma had suddenly become the naked truth of *what is* and *how it is right now*, and that "is" included me — not how I think it should be, want it to be, or long for it to be, but really how it is! I was encouraged over and over to *meet that*, until, despite all my resistance, it finally sank in.

That realization of course opened up new and often disconcerting horizons. Now I had to drop my ideas of what I thought practice and awakening looked like. We have so many wonderful mythological and inspiring examples to feed these fantasies. There are endless seductive side roads of dharma names, titles, stories of satori and "stream-entry," stories of forest monks and yogis to entertain, delight, and distract us from our real work. This or that teacher is *so* wonderful! If I could only be like them, know what they know, talk as they talk, walk as they walk. But if I were really to take on my life *as it is* as the practice of revealing both my stuckness and potential freedom, there would be nothing left to do but get serious, which means taking responsibility.

To me this assumption of responsibility means a willingness to look directly into the mirror of relationship wherever I find it, and developing the courage, endurance, and stomach to remain attentive to exactly what looks back. Looking in the mirror once or twice a day can be challenging enough, but if I take this practice seriously, I begin to find these mirrors everywhere. Indeed, if I fully commit to family life as the place and content of practice and cut off my escapes, then I discover that I'm living in a house of mirrors that continuously reflect me back to myself exactly as I am at each moment. This is a kind of intensive practice not available on silent retreats or when we view our meditation practice as limited to sitting on the cushion at particular times.

All this led to a couple of important discoveries that continue to inform how I live and teach. First, sitting meditation is a necessary but clearly not sufficient part of practice. We learn much about ourselves by showing up to meet ourselves every day in formal sitting meditation, working with a teacher, and going on retreat when possible. Sitting gives us a unique laboratory setting in which to meet and work with the "stuff" of life. We learn what it takes to have genuine intimacy with life, and what inhibits that intimacy. We can begin to dive deeply into impermanence, see how and why we suffer in the ways we do, and begin to see what this "I" is that seems to take up so much space and create such mischief in our lives. We can see that the feelings, moods, and thoughts that we call "mine" are truly aspects of every human mind. In a sense, when you've seen one mind, not only have you seen them all, you are them all, and they you.

> "I'm living in a house of mirrors that continuously reflect me back to myself exactly as I am at each moment."

This experiential understanding that I am the world and the world is me deepens intimacy with all beings and enhances that sense of responsibility as well. We can even stumble into the pristine spaciousness of awareness without the center of a "me" or an observer. In short, what we call "formal meditation practice" is really life knowing itself in the form of sitting. As thirteenth-century Zen master Dogen said, "To study Zen is to study the self." And yet again, there is so much more!

The "so much more" was the impact on my "practice" of committing to family relationships, indeed all relationships, as opportunities for awakening and liberation. J. Krishnamurti wrote that relationships reveal the ways of the self, and this is profoundly true in family life. I have never experienced the depths of fear, anger, despair, frustration, glowing joy and love, confusion and heartache, bursting pride and crushing shame to the degree and intensity that I have with my wife and daughters. Yes, I have also experienced all this deeply and intensively on the cushion and elsewhere, but not with such enduring frequency and variety.

This is not to say, of course, that this happens to everyone or that one must have a family to experience these shackles and freedoms as fully — or that "family" is defined as man, woman, kids. Family is maybe better defined as those who love me and whom I love back with commitment over time. For me this includes dear friends we have known over more than twenty-five years — couples, individuals, those with and without children. There does, however, seem to be something uniquely challenging and rewarding about working over years and years with the same intimate relationships where there are such frighteningly deep attachments and dependencies.

Then there are the developmental changes and required adaptations that occur over the life span that call for further inquiry and letting go in ever-changing permutations. Practice becomes the development of full attention to as much of this as possible, so that right in the midst of it all maybe I realize that this angry, intoxicated, coming-home-late teenager is the same child whose diapers I changed, whom I walked to her first day of school, whom I taught how to ride a bike and then drive a car, and who will eventually leave me behind for her own life's adventure. Or is it? Who is she anyway? And who am I? What does it mean to be intimate with this?!

These relationships let me know exactly and immediately where I'm stuck and where I'm free, and they beckon me to ever-deeper realms of self-knowing. It is what Dogen called the *genjokoan,* or the truth-telling place of everyday life. I can know this place with great precision because if I am willing enough and courageous enough to really listen, these people whom I love most in the world will make it very clear. They will be teaching me this truth about myself all the time.

Certainly the gaps between my dharma understanding and how I live that understanding will become increasingly clarified. Sometimes this is very good news and sometimes it's not. But it is always news. My responsibility as dharma student is to make my best effort to meet them and their news responsively and to hold self and other with the full attention that is really the essence of the healing action of spiritual practice.

So my practice has become trying to see all this as it unfolds and saying thank you if at all possible, because when it works there is an encounter of intimacy in which self and other dissolve in compassion, understanding, and lovingkindness. At those moments I know clearly both *why* and *for whom* I practice, and the gratitude for the power of practice in this interconnected web of relationship is full and spontaneous. ●

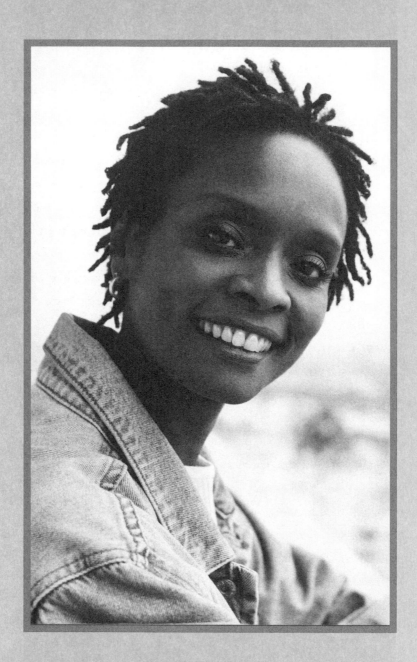

Konda Mason

NONVIOLENT ACTIVISM WITH WISDOM

KONDA MASON is the youngest of four children born to Ovaughn Marzette (lovingly known as "Kettle") and Vangle Mason. Raised in a small town in southern California, Konda attended University of California, Berkeley, where she studied rhetoric and began a lifelong involvement in the entertainment business. She directed the Berkeley Jazz Festival as an undergraduate, and later worked with the management company for the musical group Sweet Honey In The Rock in Washington, D.C. Later in New York City, Konda worked with The Creative Arts Team to bring interactive educational theater to at-risk youth. • In 1992 Konda was diagnosed with lupus, which led her to explore alternative healing modalities. She became a certified Kripalu yoga teacher and taught yoga to communities of color and at-risk youth. Konda was invited by Jack Kornfield to teach yoga at the inaugural People of Color Vipasanna Meditation Retreat in New Mexico, and continues to teach at annual retreats at Spirit Rock. She also teaches privately in Los Angeles. Konda sits on the Board of Trustees for Kripalu Center for Yoga & Health, and is a founding member of International Association of Black Yoga Teachers. • Konda's first film-producing project, the short film *Tuesday Morning Ride*, garnered her an Academy Award nomination. Her lupus is in remission.

IN THE BEGINNING WAS GOD. That was one of the only Judeo-Christian precepts that spoke to me as a child. I didn't understand much else. But every time I heard the phrase, "In the beginning was God," a feeling of absolute joy came over me. It made me feel limitless. That deep inner knowing coupled with the soul-filled gospel music of Mahalia Jackson and The Edwin Hawkins Singers constantly blaring from my mother's record player contributed to my spending the first twelve years of my life in and out of spiritual bliss.

As a child I found comfort in lying in bed with my eyes closed, listening to the early-morning sounds of birds outside my window and surrendering to the absolute feeling of joy that that connection brought me. At night it was the smell of night-blooming jasmine coming through the window that prompted the experience. Often I would fill up with so much joy that I would turn into particles of energy hovering above my bed. I would buzz around like a firefly in small packets of light energy. I remember an amazing feeling of expansion and connection. It never occurred to me to be frightened of the experience. I was always ready to go with it. I knew this special time had something to do with God and me as One. I loved the feeling these quiet times brought me. This daily ritual was my meditation practice and I craved it.

In 1967 I turned twelve and my family moved to an all-white suburb in southern California. We were the second Black family in the entire town. Painfully I experienced for the first time the world of racism and injustice. The repeated message was that I was different — that I was inferior.

That year also happens to be when my spiritual practice stopped. The connection was broken. I could no longer find the Unlimited. The dualistic world of "us" and "them" forced its way into my life and psyche. I could no longer find the "One." I spent my teenage years longing for some way to reconcile with this world filled with hatred and bigotry, as the racism in America and the war in Vietnam raged on.

As a student at UC Berkeley in the early '70s, I found my outlet in social activism. The Reagan years provided plenty of fodder for protest, but something was deeply missing at my core. I had unanswered questions about the meaning of my life.

My answer came in the form of a yogi who became an important teacher for me. He called himself Gerasimos but is now known as Raz. He was a Black man who had spent years of his life living in a Greek Orthodox monastery cooking vegetarian food and practicing yoga and meditation. I knew I wanted what he had, and he ushered me through the most profound changes in my life.

First I changed my diet and became a vegan. It was perfect for me. I realized that I had always been a vegetarian living in a carnivorous body. I immediately felt better. Next he took me to a kundalini yoga class at the 3HO house in Berkeley. The 3HO Foundation was founded by Yogi Bhajan. I had no idea who he was, but I liked the way it made me feel when I looked at his photographs. For that matter, I liked the way all the teachers looked in their white garb and turbans. They were peaceful beings and they welcomed me into their world. The name 3HO stands for Healthy, Happy, and Holy.

Through this practice of yoga, I was on my way to experiencing a healthier physical body, a deeper inner calm and focus, and my link back to the "One." My entire being soaked it up. As I lay in *savasana,* the relaxation pose at the end of class, I began to relive the experience of that expanded consciousness I had felt as a child. My heart opened wide. As I sat in meditation I felt my connection to all beings. The compassion within me swelled. It was as if the sound of the birds and the scent of the night-blooming jasmine had come back. I was home again.

So for me, spiritual practice didn't change my life; it was the absence of spiritual practice that changed it. In its absence, anger without wisdom took root. But that anger turned out to be a very important part of my journey. I needed to get mad at all the injustices of the world. And I will forever be mad about them. But through my practice of meditation and yoga, I know that true planetary healing can only happen once we stop living the myth of separation: separation of nations, separation of races, separation of classes, separation from spirit.

My passion for social, political, and economic justice for the underserved citizens of our planet is inseparable from my spiritual practice. I believe that spiritual practice must contain within it nonviolent activism with forcefulness and wisdom. My practice is not just a selfish exercise for only my personal well-being: I practice and I teach so that others may also find peace and a way out of suffering. In the words of Martin Luther King, Jr., "Justice at its best is love correcting everything that stands against love." ●

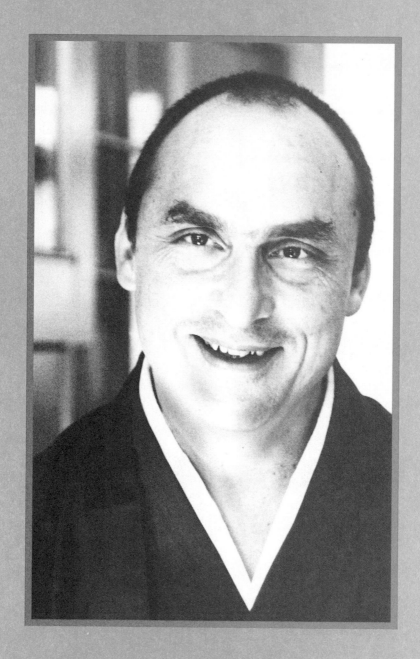

Edward Espe Brown

WHEN YOU ARE YOU, ZEN IS ZEN

EDWARD ESPE BROWN began cooking and practicing Zen in 1965 and was ordained as a priest by Shunryu Suzuki Roshi in 1971. He has been head resident teacher at each of the San Francisco Zen Centers: Tassajara, Green Gulch, and City Center, and has led meditation retreats and cooking classes throughout the United States, as well as in Austria, Germany, Spain, and England. • Ed is the author of several cookbooks, including *The Tassajara Bread Book* and *Tomato Blessing and Radish Teachings* and is the editor of *Not Always So*, a book of lectures by Shunryu Suzuki Roshi. • Ed was the first head resident cook, Tenzo, at Tassajara Zen Mountain Center, from 1967 to 1970. From 1979 to 1983 he worked at the celebrated Greens Restaurant in San Francisco, serving as busboy, waiter, floor manager, wine buyer, cashier, host, and manager. • Ed has also done extensive Vipassana practice. He has practiced yoga since 1980 and has been leading workshops and retreats with his wife, yoga teacher Patricia Sullivan, since 1988.

Q. *What kind of practice do you do these days, Ed?*

A. I start out in the morning with about forty-five minutes of Qigong and about a half hour of meditation. The rest is sort of haphazard. Sometimes I do yoga at one of my wife Patricia Sullivan's classes or someplace else, and sometimes I go to meditation retreats or lead meditation retreats.

Q. *It seems that cooking has been an important part of your practice.*

A. Absolutely, for many years. Though I haven't cooked professionally much since Tassajara, I've continued to be interested in cooking and writing cookbooks and teaching cooking classes. After I left the Zen Center it was actually the main way I supported myself for a while: teaching vegetarian cooking classes.

Q. *Is cooking part of Zen?*

A. Zen seems to be very "practical-minded." As far I can tell, Zen is what happened to Buddhism when it got to China. The Chinese are a bit more practical and down-to-earth than the Indians. They came up with all kinds of inventions early on — paper and gunpowder and what have you.

We have a sort of miniaturized Buddhist robe, this little piece of rectangular fabric with two straps that go around your neck so that it hangs in front of you. I don't think the Indians ever had that, but the Chinese didn't want to have a big cumbersome robe over their left arm and under their right shoulder, so they came up with this smaller version of Buddha's robe. They can have their hands free to do work. Monks in India weren't allowed to do work. In China they said, "A day of no work is a day of no eating."

There was an emphasis on doing something practical. Enlightenment or realization was in the doing rather than in the isolation from everything. Zen emphasizes simple things, like careful observation of the obvious. In yoga you may be carefully observing your body and your posture and your breath. In meditation you're observing your posture and your breath and your mind, and focusing on being present. I tell people in cooking class: "Now taste what you put in your mouth." That's pretty basic, but not so different from "Feel your feet" or "Notice your inhalation and exhalation" or what have you.

Q. *So you teach mindfulness in cooking?*

A. Yes. The other thing I emphasize besides mindfulness is joy, enjoyment, savoring. Why not enjoy and delight in food and cooking and eating, rather than worry about whether it's good enough or you're eating just the right thing — whether you're eating this and not eating that, and it's good for you or it's bad for you, or if you're sitting or you're not, or you're feeling guilty. There are so many weird things about food.

I'm convinced that if you actually enjoy what you're eating and taste what you put in your mouth, your diet will change. Mine does. Then you don't have to discipline yourself. I've done the "eat just one potato chip" test. People say things like, "Gee, there was an instant of salt and grease and then a tasteless pulp in my mouth. I would have gone on eating more, trying to get what I didn't get the first time, if I hadn't realized that that's just the way it is."

If you're mindful and present, you realize that this potato chip experience isn't that interesting or enjoyable. Or, if it is enjoyable, then after an ounce or so of chips, you might say, "OK, that's enough. It was good but it's not good anymore." Rather than trying to behave according to some program, you're actually mindful and responding to your own experience, awake enough to make good, clear choices, or so-called wise choices.

Q. *So you don't eat a pound of potato chips at a time?*

A. I don't do mindless eating. I created my own diet plan, and last fall I found out my diet plan is the same as Julia Child's diet plan. Her diet plan, it turns out, is small portions, no seconds, eat widely, enjoy yourself. The main thing I had to do was slow down and then begin to notice the difference between enjoyment and when enjoyment goes over to excitement or greed or lust.

Enjoyment is when you're actually having a sense of ease or calm that goes along with the pleasure, and there's not the sense of grasping and trying to get more while you still have food in your mouth.

Q. *Was cooking your first practice?*

A. I started meditating, going to the Zen Center in San Francisco in May of 1965. That was also when I started cooking. I had lived a little bit on my own before, but that's when I really was living on my own and somehow was more drawn to cooking. I found out that I enjoyed it.

I had been struggling. I went to college for a year at Antioch and dropped out in 1964 because school wasn't satisfying. For instance, I took a social psychology course where I wrote a paper about "Alienation and Anxiety." At the end I was just as alienated and anxious as ever, even though I got an "A" on the paper. It just seemed really impractical to me.

I wanted to find something in my life that was very practical. I also thought it would be good just to sit still and be quiet. I found a group of people who were doing that — just sitting still. I couldn't sit still without having a group of people to sit with. I'd sit down and after a minute I'd get up and turn on the stereo or have a cup of coffee or open a book.

I had the sense that "Gee, I don't want to be just a slave to whatever happens to pop into my mind next." What kind of life is that? You know, something occurs to you that you could do that supposedly is going to make some difference and make you happier, and it's just something else to do. I haven't noticed over the years that that's particularly effective, and practicing Zen has been helpful in letting go of compulsive behaviors, or at least awakening the capacity to choose.

Q. *Was meditation difficult for you to start with? Was it difficult for you to sit for long periods?*

A. Well, yes and no. For one forty-minute period it wasn't so difficult, but the Zen people like to sit all day for days on end. So as soon as I started sitting for two or three periods it was extremely difficult; it was painful.

I had a very important experience early on. I had started gritting my teeth and grimacing and I was hardly breathing. Sitting next to me was a woman named Jean Ross, who was, at the time, the president of Zen Center. She'd actually practiced Zen in Japan — a great, older woman, she was in her sixties then. She reached over and put her hand on my knee.

People never do that — never touch anybody else in meditation. You let everybody else do his or her own practice. But it was very matter-of-fact. The curious thing about her touch was that she wasn't giving me any directive — it was just touch and presence.

It ended up being very calming. After a while, not only did the pain disappear, my body basically disappeared, and there was just this glow there. Then I could feel the outlines of my body coming back and pretty soon she took her hand away. That helped me. I used to feel her hand there from time to time after that.

I'd had the idea that a lot of what happens in life is just your mind, as opposed to what's happening. And that was an experience of something like that. But sitting got more and more and more difficult, and my particular experience of it was not only pain; I also had involuntary movements for about two years.

Q. *What was that like?*

A. My head would jerk back and forth, or my whole body would shake. I'd try to stop my head from jerking back and forth and then my body would start shaking. Any place I tried to hold onto and stop from moving, the movement would just be someplace else.

From time to time Suzuki Roshi used to come around and put his hands on my shoulders and that was very calming, similar to what had happened with Jean Ross. But they didn't know whether I should go on sitting or not. Sometimes I'd have to sit in the entryway to the meditation hall instead of in the meditation hall proper. I would relax, then I'd fall asleep. In those days, if you fell asleep, someone would hit you. So it was either wake up and shake or go to sleep and get hit. It was extremely traumatic.

There was a period when we were doing a week of meditation and in the afternoon of the third day I just gave up because I was getting hit three or four times a period and shaking. Kobun Chino was there. He came and said, "Let's go outside." Crossing e threshold of the door, I started sobbing. He led me back to my room. I couldn't see anything I was sobbing so much. He had me lie down on the bed, and then he started sort of massaging me. I was sobbing without restraint and my arms and legs were flapping uncontrollably.

Q. *Ed, why did you keep sitting?*

A. It's hard to know. I think of it as faith — and knowing Suzuki Roshi. My relationship with him was very important. Thich Nhat Hanh talks about how you have a birth family, or blood family, and a spiritual family. That was very definitely like having a spiritual family as well as a blood family — having another father. It was just amazing.

I'm not the only one who felt that way; I think many people felt that Suzuki Roshi could see through you and it was "no problem," which was quite refreshing compared with the usual thought "If anybody knew who I really am, they would hate me the way I hate myself." You may have that sort of worry about your spiritual teachers, or whoever your partner is, but I felt seen and known and loved, and I felt that I was actually OK. Kobun Chino was like that for me, too. He wasn't that much older than I was so he was a little bit more like an older brother to me.

I also felt rather estranged from everybody, and once in a while people would get mad at me, saying, "You're just doing that for attention" and "You could stop those movements if you really wanted to" and blah, blah, blah: "It's not really involuntary" and "What's your problem?" and "Why don't you just calm down?" I keep finding out that I am just a very intensely emotional person. You can spend your life trying not to be and it doesn't help. I also had a very traumatic childhood.

Q. *It sounds as though your nervous system was unwinding itself.*

A. That's as good a description as any, I suppose. People I know who have involuntary movements seem to be, like me, fairly high strung. There's a reason why you're tightly wired, which is so that you won't feel the intensely painful feelings that otherwise you might. Simple enough.

Q. *But a lot of it is probably also precognitive trauma that meditation actually reaches.*

A. Suzuki Roshi's encouragement was to acknowledge your weak point rather than hiding it; otherwise you could spend your whole life hiding your weak point. His teaching was to acknowledge it and be real, or be human, rather than aiming to be perfect or act according to some standard that you have in mind. He talks about this in *Not Always So,* a book of his lectures that I edited. "Express yourself," he says. "Expose yourself . . . especially to your teacher." He also mentions that "the purpose of practice and training" is not "just to correct your weak points," because then "it would be almost impossible to succeed. Even so, it is necessary to work on them, because as you work on them, your character will be trained, and you will become free of ego."

One of my favorite lines of his was when we were right in the middle of a seven-day *sesshin* [intensive meditation retreat]. It was either the third or fourth morning. He started his talk, and shortly into it he said: "The problems you are now experiencing . . ." and I thought "are just temporary, are delusion." He said "will continue . . ." and I thought "until you understand better." Then he said "will continue for the rest of your life." We all laughed. There was something about the way he said that. He had that sort of subtle, droll humor.

We were all waiting for him to say "The problems you are now experiencing are just temporary." There's something very true about that, and there's also something about how much easier life is, actually, if you're not all the time bemoaning the fact that the problems are still there. You just have them. There's knowing that and then there's actually living it. I keep reminding myself, because otherwise it's easy to be upset that the problems are still continuing.

Q. *So meditation has helped you be more comfortable with who you are?*

A. Suzuki Roshi's expression, which I liked very much — I think it was probably in *Zen Mind, Beginner's Mind* — was "When you are you, Zen is Zen." When you start out doing spiritual practice you think you're going to become Zen, become better than you.

W. S. Merwin had a poem "To Waiting" in which he's talking about how you are waiting to become someone even better than you. It's really quite wonderful. Of course while you are waiting to become somebody even better, you miss your life. It's a poetic expression of Suzuki Roshi's reminder that when you seek for improvement, you lose your present life.

Rather than becoming Zen or enlightened or whatever, you become *you* — and finally it's OK to be you. It's interesting how much courage and commitment it takes, and that's part of what was so amazing about Suzuki Roshi, his capacity to give permission and support for each person to be who he or she is, not trying to measure up to some standard or ideal but just to be themselves. That's how I now understand realization or enlightenment or awakening. Enlightenment is really deep trust in yourself, and when you're resting in this trust, your life just unfolds.

Your being you is an expression of the divine or what's beyond. For you to be you, you're letting what is beyond come through you and manifest in your life. It's not exactly that it's yours. It's just coming through you. You are "practicing" enlightenment, and people say, "Thank you for being you." ●

TO WAITING

You spend so much of your time
expecting to become
someone else
always someone
who will be different
someone to whom a moment
whatever moment it may be
at last has come
and who has been
met and transformed
into no longer being you
and so has forgotten you

meanwhile in your life
you hardly notice
the world around you
lights changing
sirens dying along the buildings
your eyes intent
on a sight you do not see yet
not yet there
as long as you
are only yourself

with whom as you
recall you were
never happy
to be left alone for long

— W. S. MERWIN

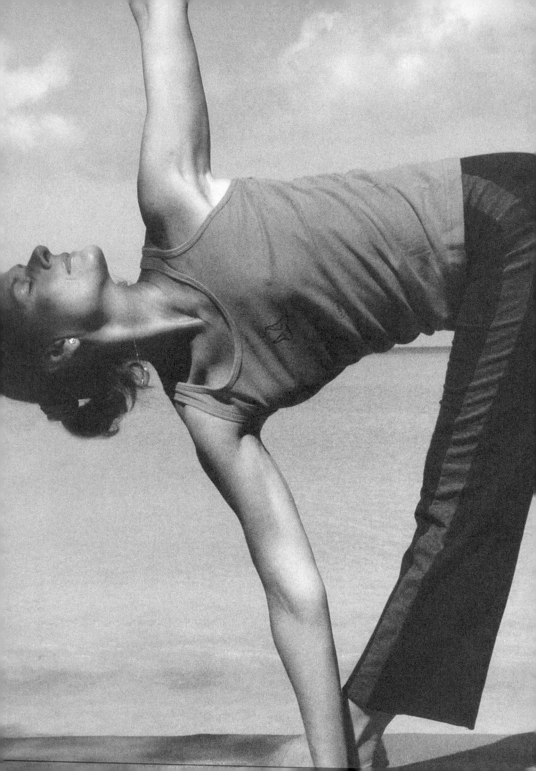

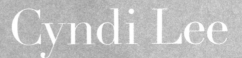

Cyndi Lee

PRACTICING TO SAVE MY LIFE

CYNDI LEE founded OM yoga center in New York City in 1998. Her first yoga class was in college in 1972. After completing her graduate thesis on women, dance, and spirituality at the University of Calfornia, Irvine, Cyndi arrived in New York on an Art History Fellowship to the Whitney Museum of American Art. This was a wonderful opportunity to learn but not enough cash, so Cyndi began teaching yoga in Greenwich Village. Soon she became a fixture in the downtown modern dance scene, choreographing and performing primarily in XXY Dance/Music and Cyndi Lee Dance Company/Big Moves, Inc. Cyndi also choreographed over twenty music videos including Cyndi Lauper's "Girls Just Want to Have Fun." • After meeting her root guru, Gelek Rinpoche, in the late 1980s, Cyndi's practice of yoga and Buddhism merged with her choreography. In 1994, "Dharma Dances" was her last concert, which featured Allen Ginsberg singing his own songs and accompanying himself on harmonium. • Cyndi is the author and illustrator of *OM Yoga: A Guide to Daily Practice; OM at Home: A Yoga Journal; OM Yoga in a Box* series; and *Yoga Body, Buddha Mind* (Riverhead Books 2004). She has written for *Tricycle, Dance Magazine, BalletTanz, Spa Finder, Cooking Light,* and has a regular column in *Shambhala Sun,* and writes the *vinyasa* column for *Yoga Journal.*

IT CAME WITHOUT WARNING right at the beginning of the day-trip down the river. I really don't like water and I'm a weak swimmer, but people I trusted said the trip would be fun and not that scary. They assured me that if you fell out of the boat, you would land on a little rock and immediately be picked up by the next boat. So I went along, and after the very first bend in the river, I slid out.

There was no warning and no big inhale before I was accidentally plunged into icy cold, wildly churning water. There I was, trapped under a rubber boat in the white-water rapids of the Pacuare River in Costa Rica.

No breath in my lungs and nobody able to see where I was, I thought, "Wow, this is how it happens." I visualized a small article in *The New York Times:* "Yoga Teacher Drowns while Leading Retreat in Costa Rica." My mind raced and my lungs got tight, but somehow I didn't panic. The yoga and meditation practices I had been doing for years prepared me for that moment.

Pranayama — manipulation and retention of the breath — helped me know intuitively that I could go without breath longer than was comfortable. Asana — my daily twisting and inverting — enabled me to know what was up and down and to maintain a highly fluid sense of balance. Meditation — my daily practice of training my mind — let me keep my focus on the task at hand, even while thoughts of my own death ran rampant through my head. After groping my way along the bottom of the boat, I finally popped up into the rapids.

A very long minute later, a bodybuilder/yoga student floated by, grabbed me by the collar, and plopped me into his boat. Gelek

Rinpoche, a Tibetan lama, had taught me that to meet the dharma in your life is as fortunate and rare as a tortoise's head popping up in an inner tube in the middle of the ocean. In that moment I felt like that tortoise.

Sitting in the haven of "boat number two," my heart hammering, my adrenaline rushing, my lungs gasping, I was as scared as I'd ever been. Under the boat I had not been scared. I had been wide awake, balanced, and steady. Mindfulness meditation, yoga asanas, and *pranayama* are all powerful practices that can affect us deeply, but there is no doubt in my mind that in that life-threatening moment, it was the combination of all three that saved my life.

Back in 1972 I started taking yoga classes for easy physical education credit in college. The feeling of being cleansed, soothed, and stretched was unmatched by any other type of exercise I had experienced. My teachers were inspiring and I was highly motivated. It didn't take long for me to be able to hold my breath for over a minute, or stand on my head for five minutes. However, my experience with the physical practice of yoga was not enough for me. I had an empty feeling and a longing for something more.

Remembering that my dad's prescription for "the blahs" was to do something helpful for someone else, I searched for a way to take the focus off myself and began to explore *maitri,* the lovingkindness aspect of Tibetan Buddhism. When a friend of mine invited me to attend a two-week intensive retreat with His Holiness the Dalai Lama, I went eagerly.

Some of the teachers wore business suits; some wore elaborate robes. I didn't have a clue who they were or what they said, but I liked being there. In the second week, when the Dalai Lama explained what it meant to be a *bodhisattva,* a person who dedicates her life to helping others, I took the vow without hesitation.

At the time of my introduction to Buddhism, I was already a passionate student of yoga, and I've been fortunate to have shared yoga with my own students over the past twenty years. Now I've been a student of Tibetan Buddhism for more than twelve years, and the two traditions have come together in my teaching. The teachings of yoga and Buddhism complement each other and together form a basic homework assignment for humans: what to do with this body and this mind.

Have yoga and meditation changed my life? Very much so. The most profound benefit of yoga and meditation for me has been a natural relaxing into my life. Obstacles are not so scary. I am more fluid, more curious, and at the same time more patient. I have more options for happiness because I don't require specific conditions.

It is a relief to discover that I can be happy even if the world doesn't revolve around me or my agenda. This has opened me to other people. I want others to be happy, which sometimes brings a feeling of sadness as well as sweetness. In other words, practice has allowed me to be a real human being.

During the summer before my first marriage broke up, I cried a lot in yoga class. When we lay down for the final relaxation, tears would pour out of my eyes, almost as if I were leaking. This went on every day for the whole summer. Somehow the release of effort in my muscles and toxins in my organs led to the release of emotions in my heart and mind.

As I embodied my sadness more and more, it traveled out of me, and by the end of the summer I felt clean, balanced, and brave enough to make the necessary changes. It turned out that even though it was painful, my summer of being heartbroken was better than having no heart at all.

According to Chogyam Trungpa, "The way to rule the universe is to expose your heart." When the ebb and flow of our heart diminishes, we feel separate from the vast world around us in which everything breathes and pulsates, expands and contracts.

My experience has been that when my heart is broken, just as in my summer of tears, my boundaries start to soften and dissolve. When my father was told that he needed to have brain surgery, we realized he might not live long. Our small family — my mom, dad, and I — were shaken and frightened, yet I have never felt so alive as I did during the time of his surgery.

We had no idea what would happen. Everything was extremely intense and vivid. On the operating table the doctors discovered that my father had a serious brain infection but no tumor. Daddy would survive and be okay. During that period I practiced *maitri* meditation for him every day. When I first saw that big Frankenstein's monster-like scar on his head, my instinctive response was to touch my own head. In that moment I felt no separation between my head and his, my heart and his.

Life always manages to bring one obstacle or another. I

understand that now and I don't resist it as much. Practice for me is no longer about getting *rid* of obstacles, but learning to *relate* to them creatively.

Recently I had an "aha" while watching the weather report on television. The reporter was explaining that when the wind from the north and the Gulf Stream come together in a certain way, the result is more snow in New York City! Usually I ignored that part of the weather report and just waited to be briefed so that I could plan my next day's outfit. Suddenly I realized that weather is like yoga practice. It's all about conditions coming together and the possible outcomes that can result.

After many years of practice I think of yoga as a process of understanding myself and others through the vehicle of my body. Watching my body move in and out of energetic and neurological patterns with purposeful attention is similar to what a weather reporter does with the weather. By paying close attention to my body, mind, and breath, I have learned to recognize the different patterns that arise (e.g., this grouping will create rain) and then make appropriate choices (I need an umbrella). I don't know in advance what will actually manifest, but choosing to be open, patient, and fascinated by life's events is what carries me through.

I always come back to *vinyasa:* the notion that one thing flows into another. One thing arises, then dissolves as the next thing arises, then dissolves. Having gradually recognized the nature of my life and of all life, I now have more confidence and composure to rest in a state of not knowing. ●

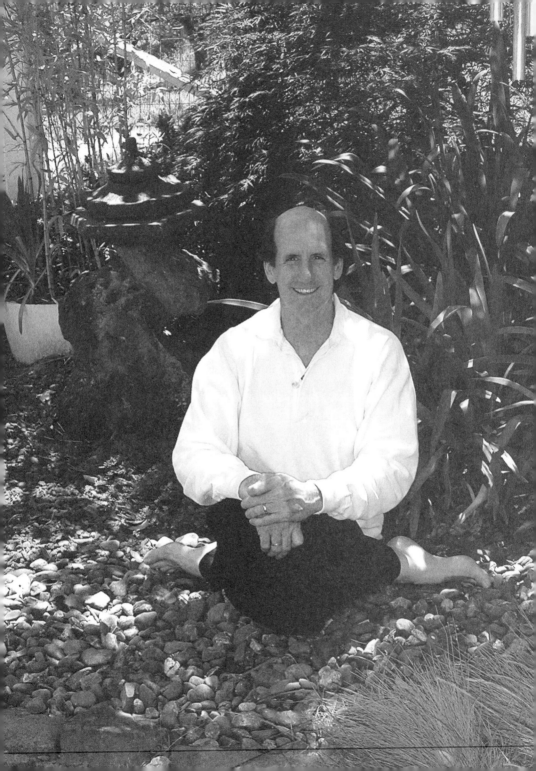

Richard Miller

THE SEARCH FOR ONENESS

RICHARD MILLER has followed the path of nondualism ever since the universe revealed its truth of oneness as he gazed into the night sky at the age of thirteen. Along the way he studied Taoism and Chinese medicine, coauthored *The Book of Internal Exercises*, and volunteered his acupuncture skills at a village clinic while studying yoga in India. He holds a B.S. in psychology, an M.A. in communication, and a Ph.D. in clinical psychology. • Richard's teachers include Laura Cummings, T. K. V. Desikachar, Ramesh Balsekar, and Suzanne Segal. It was while studying with his spiritual mentor, Jean Klein, that all sense of separation fell away. Richard experiences this awakening as always fresh, alive, and opening to itself. In private practice since 1972, he continues working with people interested in awakening. • Richard has been honored by *Yoga Journal* and featured in the book *American Yoga*. He cofounded the International Association of Yoga Therapy and was founding editor of its professional journal. He has authored numerous articles including "Welcoming All That Is," in Paragon's *The Sacred Mirror: Nondual Wisdom and Psychotherapy*. He is writing two books on meditation. Richard enjoys hosting retreats where people gather to experience his creative way of teaching individual, interpersonal and impersonal, dimensions of Self.

"When the Guest is being searched for, it is the intensity of the desire that does all the work. Look at me, and you will see a slave of that intensity."

— KABIR

Q. *How has practice changed your life, Richard?*

A. Originally I hoped that practice would end my suffering once and for all. I imagined attaining a perfected state of body and mind where there would never be pain again. What I found was very different. In 1976 I was practicing the King Dancer's Pose, holding my leg behind my head while standing balanced on the opposite leg. I asked myself, "What have I attained after so much effort?" I realized that were I to walk out the door and be hit by a car, the flexibility I had gained would be worthless. At that moment I realized that the goal of hatha yoga had to be more than the attainment of some perfected body position. And that has been true ever since.

Q. *What would you say are the goals of practice?*

A. In my experience the goal of practice is different for each person. We are each facets of unity. Each of us is an expression of oneness, the mysterious vastness that is the home ground of everything. It is apparent that vastness wants to experience itself in every possible manner: as the person searching and realizing enlightenment and as the person searching and not realizing it; as the person suffering and as the person realizing an end to suffering.

For me, however, the goal of practice has always been bringing an end to suffering. Until enlightenment there was always incompleteness and doubt plaguing my mind. The feeling of incompleteness and doubt are gone now, replaced with an ineffable peace and aliveness that I could never have imagined, yet always thought was possible.

Yoga practice has made the body/mind sensitive to the slightest movement of the mind away from our inherent spontaneity. This has brought with it skillfulness in communicating in relationship. And it has brought fearlessness, so that every experience, emotion, and thought is allowed into consciousness without the attitude of suppression that dominated my prior life. I feel a responsiveness and integrity in all my relationships, in work, and in friendships with all people.

Returning to the goals — practice has had two important and interrelated goals for me throughout the years: first, the purification and cleansing of the body/mind, and second, a gradual immersion in non-separative consciousness. From early childhood I sought to heal an inner sense of estrangement and a feeling of separation and bewilderment.

I remember the actual moment it began: I was two years old. To my right was the doorway and to my left a window looking out onto the lawn. As I moved toward the doorway, suddenly everything was present, the door, the window with the light coming through it, and my sister standing in front of me. In that moment I realized that I was separate from her. Until that moment I had had no self-consciousness; now I was aware of everything as distinct and separate from me.

Over the years no amount of talking with others or working it out on my own helped resolve this inner conflict of separation, but it led me to pursue many practices that touched upon or combined yoga, meditation, psychology, and medicine. Throughout my search, however, meditative self-inquiry always remained the pivotal experience.

Q. *What traditions have served as the source of your practice?*

A. My tradition has been the path of unqualified nondualism as reflected through the teachings of Kashmir Shaivism, Advaita, and Dzogchen. I was also intrigued by the Gnostic teachings of Christianity, mystical Judaism, Sufism, Taoism, and Zen. In all these teachings, ego is seen as a projection of the mind and is inherently empty of substance. The teachings inform us that separation is a false belief that gives rise to suffering, which in turn is a messenger calling us back to heal this moment of separation. When our false sense of separation dissolves, we discover that our true underlying nature is an always-present equanimity that is saturated with peace, openness, and unqualified joy.

Q. *How did you first get involved in yoga practice?*

A. I had moved to California after getting my B.S. in psychology. After reading an article on yoga, I attended my first class at the Integral Yoga Institute in San Francisco. At the end of the lesson the instructor led us through *yoga nidra,* which entailed paying attention to opposing experiences within the body, such as tension-relaxation, warmth-coolness, and agitation-calmness. I was invited to rotate my attention through each pair of opposites until I was able to embody each opposing experience while containing its opposite.

That evening I drove home feeling expansively present and alive, radiant and joyful. I experienced life in its perfection and my "self" as spacious, nonlocalized presence. While the experience slowly faded over the next several weeks, it left a deep longing to awaken consciously into and fully abide in that presence.

Q. *What other experiences affected your practice?*

A. Occasionally and unpredictably throughout my life, just as in that first class in San Francisco, I experienced shifts in consciousness where I suddenly felt present and free of conflict, attuned with the whole universe. Most of the time it happened while out in nature.

At the age of thirteen I spent Easter vacation with my grandmother in Florida. She always wanted me to attend the local dances. To placate her I'd go along, but usually entered the front door only to walk out the back. Often I'd take a walk with a thirteen-year-old friend of mine, and we'd end up gazing together into the nighttime sky. One evening we had walked along the nearby golf course and settled down in a sand trap by the eighth green. Looking up at the heavens, I started wondering where the end of the universe was.

In my mind I was traveling through it until I came to a brick wall. Then suddenly I jumped up and over this wall, and I was again traveling until I encountered another brick wall. But again my knowing had me jump over that wall, and the next and the next, until suddenly I was flooded with this feeling of endlessness and vastness. I knew then, without doubt, that the cosmos had no beginning and no end. I also knew that I was not separate from the totality of this cosmos.

Glimpses like these were invariably short-lived, leaving me melancholy and bewildered. How could I obtain such a radical understanding and have it endure? Years later, after the experience of my first yoga class, I recognized that yoga could be a portal through which I could realize my longing for freedom from separation and conflict.

Shortly after moving to San Francisco I began volunteering at the San Francisco Suicide Prevention Center, where I learned to intervene with people in psychological or drug-related crises. Later I also began volunteering at a local clinic, where I trained the staff in those same crisis-intervention skills. During a discussion about the training with one of the clinic's supervising psychotherapists, Laura Cummings, the two of us recognized how working together might serve both our needs — mine to be trained in the art of psychotherapy and hers as a supervisor needing students.

For the next five years I sat in with Laura during every one of her psychotherapy sessions. At the end of our first session working together, Laura invited me to tell her what I had experienced during the session. After relating to her all that I had observed, she inquired, "Yes, but what happened inside you?" Thus began my real training.

Q. *What skills did you learn through that mentorship?*

A. In my work with Laura and through my daily hatha yoga and meditation, I learned the skill of tracking subtle movements of sensation, thought, and feeling within my clients and myself. Psychology and spirituality began to merge as two movements that intimately supported and enriched each other. Psychology was teaching me how to be with every movement of life, while meditative inquiry was teaching me how to be the container of mysterious vastness out of which, within which, and back into which every movement of life unfolded.

One evening while talking with Laura, I suddenly had the experience of being at one with the universe, feeling no separation either within myself or with any outer object. This was the strongest glimpse of true nature that I had ever experienced. It lasted for several weeks and left behind a deep knowing that complete freedom from suffering was possible.

During my studies of yoga I had read about the experience of enlightenment that culminated in the steady abiding in a state of Unity Consciousness. It occurred to me that if enlightenment was possible, it had to be possible for everyone, including myself, as it was the realization of true nature that we all share in common. With that understanding in place, I earnestly dedicated myself to embodying and realizing that aim.

Q. *What other teachers influenced you?*

A. In 1979 I was invited to study with T. K. V. Desikachar in India and under his tutelage learned Ayurvedic principles of yoga as well as sutra and chanting. I continued working closely with him from 1980 until 1985, even helping to found Viniyoga America, an organization to further his teachings in the West.

Mentoring with Desikachar was, for me, a coming home into a lineage that supported all that I had learned through my years of study. I spent many years integrating his unique approach, adapting yoga to the individual. I also began graduate studies in marital and family therapy in 1982, and finished my Ph.D. in clinical psychology in 1987. In addition to working in private practice as a psychotherapist and teaching weekly yoga classes, I wrote articles for *Yoga Journal* and other magazines and traveled throughout the United States offering seminars and retreats.

Of course marriage and family have been profound teachers for me. In 1981 I married my wife, whom I had met at the Mill Valley Holistic Health Institute, where I gave noontime talks on yoga and meditation. We are happily celebrating our twenty-second anniversary in 2003 and live with our children in Sonoma County, California. I feel tremendous gratitude for our relationship and for the mutual interest in communication that has supported our spiritual growth over the years.

Just last week we were having a conversation about how my practice has affected our relationship. Suddenly my wife turned to me and said, "You know, you feel very impersonal these days. I could be just anybody to you." While I acknowledged that it was true, I also informed her of the fact that it is she that I love and want to come home to each night. Love, to me, is a mystery to be lived. I can't say why I love her, I just do. Over the years, we've developed a very deep understanding and resonance with one another. We both understand that conflict is rooted in ego, and whenever there's conflict between us, we rise to the challenge immediately. As well, I am grateful for my children, my associates, and my friends, as each relationship has encouraged my spiritual and psychological growth.

Of all my teachers, however, Jean Klein stands out as the spiritual mentor who pointed me directly to the ultimate truth of being. In 1983 I met Jean, an enlightened teacher of unqualified nondualism. In my first meeting with him I felt that I had finally come home to the teacher and teachings I had been waiting for all my life. Jean's teachings were a direct pointer to true nature as unqualified vastness in which everything is whole and unified.

One day Jean said to me, "Your very trying to change yourself is actually taking you away from what you are." In other words, my very search for enlightenment was keeping me trapped in a separate self. I took Jean's words to heart, and self-inquiry became the 24/7 practice that kept me probing the depths of my being on a moment-to-moment basis. It became apparent that the mind's holding to its beliefs lay at the heart of separation and suffering. Each time I had a glimpse of true nature I could feel myself not as ego, but as openness that deconstructed all sense of being separate. I began to experience how thought was a movement that arose in me, but I was the openness in which that movement occurred.

One night in 1996, after not being able to fall asleep, I got up and sat by the door, looking out at the backyard. It must have been three o'clock in the morning. All of a sudden my perspective shifted and all sense of separation fell away. In one remarkable moment I knew who I was as the vastness itself, empty yet full, open, timeless and without center or periphery. In that moment there were no bells or whistles, just the tacit understanding that everything is one ineffable unitive substance and I am that. The understanding arose that everything is empty of "self" because everything is not separate from anything else. Tremendous gratitude and joyous thanks welled up in me for all the teachers who helped me along the way, as well as for all the struggles that I had endured that had delivered me to this timeless moment.

Interestingly, nagging doubts continued to arise for several years in relation to this awakening. The ego struggles with itself. But the ego is a mirage of the mind, a projected belief based on memory. This belief has been reinforced over decades, lifetimes. Even though we realize the fundamental truth of our timeless vastness, residues of belief continue to arise and eliminate. But there came a moment for me when truth affirmed itself without the need of an external teacher and these lingering doubts dissolved.

Q. *And how would you describe what happened in that moment?*

A. As I developed my yoga and self-inquiry practice and opened into the experience of "no self," my suffering completely vanished. Pain and the difficulties of life continue to be experienced, but without the mind's interference, without wanting things to be different. The irony that I could never have imagined is that there is no "self" to enjoy the experience; there is simply joy and experiencing, but no experiencer.

Last week my wife was giving me feedback about something I had done, and I could immediately feel my defenses rising. However, as old residues of defense arise, they're immediately seen and witnessed, and in that same process dismantled. There's no place for separation; it keeps getting undone as it arises. Before it used to take days or weeks. Now it's down to seconds and minutes.

Whenever my mind begins to split from its underlying ground of oneness, sensations arise such as discomfort and anxiety to signal that the mind is entertaining some belief of separation. Splitting is registered as a bodily cue of sensation. Hatha yoga, *pranayama,* and meditation have sensitized me to these cues.

I often think of Buddha's conversations with Ananda, his attendant. Greeting him in the morning, the Buddha was reported at times to have said one of two things, "Last night Mara came and visited me. I saw who it was and he immediately went on his way." Or, "Last night Mara came. I invited him in and we had tea and a very long chat." What that means is that sometimes we release struggle automatically and sometimes we must sit with it until the worn-out thought-forms depart. Awakening doesn't bring an end to the mind's residue; past conditioning and patterned thinking still erupt from time to time, but the difference is that now we invite them in for a cup of tea.

Q. *Do you feel your practice affects others as well as yourself?*

A. I feel certain that the change wrought by my practice also changes the world. I don't see how it can be otherwise. Everything is interconnected in the fabric of oneness. Awakening affects the entire world. I don't need to change the world. When I don't go away from myself, when I live my true nature and feel myself as total peace in each moment, this has a tremendous effect on the entire universe.

I imagine myself as a piece of cloth that's been repeatedly dyed and left in the sun to dry. After repeated exposures to the dye and sun, the color no longer fades. That's the way I feel about my practice; abiding in the unqualified vastness of true nature has rendered me colorfast. ●

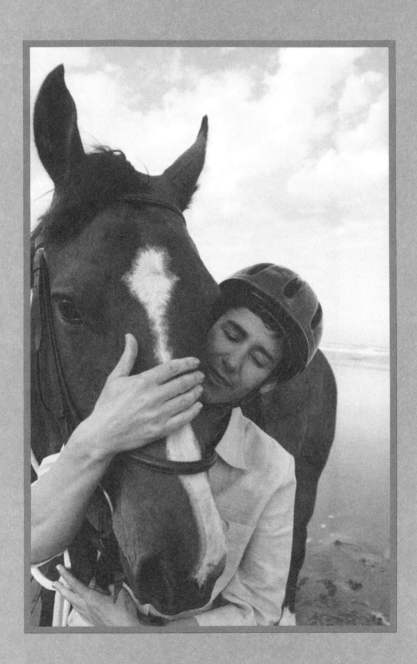

Donna Farhi

PAYING ATTENTION

DONNA FARHI is a yoga teacher who has been practicing for twenty-nine years and teaching for more than twenty years. She leads intensives, retreats, and teacher-training programs internationally. Trained initially as a dancer and then as a yoga teacher, Donna became disillusioned with practices that focused almost exclusively upon the attainment of form, recognizing that when we strive to become "some body" we often negate and refuse the "some one" that we are in the moment. For years she has been inquiring with her beloved students into the question of who we are and what is possible when we drop all concepts, ideas, techniques, and embellishments. As a result of her discoveries, she wrote the now contemporary classic *The Breathing Book* and later followed with *Yoga Mind, Body & Spirit: A Return to Wholeness*, in which she focuses on the refinement of the universal movement principles that underlie all yoga practice. • Donna has been the asana columnist for *Yoga Journal* and *Yoga International Magazine (U.S.A)*. Her third book, *Bringing Yoga to Life: The Everyday Practice of Enlightened Living,* is an exploration of yoga as a lifelong apprenticeship. American-born, Donna now resides in Christchurch, New Zealand, where she indulges her passion for horses.

Q. *How has yoga transformed your life, Donna?*

A. I think the most palpable difference is that previously I would have said that I experience the universe as a fundamentally hostile, frightening place. That was quite a dominant experience for me as a child, and certainly well into my twenties and early thirties. You could say that throughout the better part of my life I experienced change as threatening.

My experience now is that the universe is basically a friendly place and I have a new sense of fearlessness in relationship to life. Somehow yoga has helped me give birth to an immense trust in life that I didn't have before. Certainly fear still arises for me, but it's now what I would call a secondary experience — whereas before, my primary experience was this fearfulness.

Practice for me has been about shifting my perspective so that my primary experience is the ground — that which essentially is uninjured, has never been hurt, and never can be hurt. I'm qualifying it because when enlightenment is put forward as a state of fearlessness, or a state of being beyond being hurt, there can be a misunderstanding, thinking that we never feel again, we never have a moment when we get angry or feel jealousy or any of those sorts of so-called negative emotions. It's rather that they become secondary and are witnessed from this other place: the ground. This is much more than a theoretical understanding for me. It's very much a direct, lived thing.

It is a great relief, I must say, after living the better part of my life in a state of paralyzing terror. A huge part of my fear as a child and young adult was that I was going to be moved. This was not an idle or imagined fear. My father moved the family a lot and I lived in a state of anxiety that any day my father was going to come home and announce that we were going to move to some strange place and I'd be uprooted once again. My father still has wanderlust. At one point he was actually talking about moving the family to New Guinea, so you can imagine what the mind of a child might do with that looming possibility.

It's truly ironic that now virtually half my life is spent as an itinerant yoga teacher — constantly moving around, going into countries I've never been to before, sometimes even placing myself in potentially dangerous situations.

Q. *Were you aware of this pervasive fear state when you started doing yoga?*

A. I was consciously aware that I was frightened. As a child I even feared for myself physically because as an American I was swept into the equivalent of a ghetto school where I was living in New Zealand. There was tremendous aggression toward foreigners in the '70s. For instance, another young girl at my school had been put over a barbed-wire fence on the way home simply because she was a foreigner. So I really feared for my physical safety often in just going to school. My parents were unfortunately unaware that that was going on, so I was very alone with it.

What was remarkable to me about my first yoga class at school when I was sixteen was that I felt — for just a brief moment of time — completely safe. Safe! And that safety felt so precious. I discovered that I could conjure up that same feeling through practicing yoga by myself at home. So my love for yoga was instantaneous. I had my first class and from Day One I was practicing at home for an hour every day after school. I would go up to my room and practice asanas and some *pranayama* and meditation.

Q. *So the yoga mat was a safe place for you from the beginning?*

A. Right from the first class. The very first practice that I did, I thought, "Wow, I actually have some control over this experience. I can create a safe place for myself." I don't think it was on a conscious level. When you're sixteen you don't think, "Ah, I'm going to go into my room to create a safe place for myself." But there was something that drew me like a magnet to practice. While at the time it seemed quite ordinary, looking back now as a teacher, it's very unusual to have a sixteen-year-old come to class, and even more unusual for them to be practicing of their own volition at home.

Q. *Do you think that you learned early on in your practice to cue yourself into an altered state? An equanimous state?*

A. I am totally uninterested in altered states because basically I think we're in an altered state all the time. We're altered in that we're living in a kind of *distorted reality* all the time. What I'm looking for when I'm on my mat is that which is *not* distorted, that which *isn't* altered. I think the concern with altered states is more or less the conundrum people get into in practice. They think that when they do yoga they're going to have this really high, altered, pure, out-of-body experience.

I get a lot of letters from people who talk about wanting — or having had — an out-of-body experience, asking, "How can I keep having those?" I'll say, "Why on earth would you want to be even more in an altered state, because that's the problem!" The problem is that we're in an altered state all the time. So I look for a very simple experience on the mat, simply noticing the altered state of distraction and busyness, and witnessing it. I would say that as much as the mat is a refuge for me, it can also be a place of confrontation.

Q. *Can you say more about how the mat has been a place of confrontation for you?*

A. I'll give you an example that's very close to my heart at the moment. It was a time when I noticed a distinct and palpable shift in my practice. It was when my brother Robert was dying and during the year after he died. I would go to the mat and, of course, as happens when any of us enters this practice space, I would become more available to whatever was my dominant experience. At the time of my brother's illness and death, my dominant experience was deep sadness. There was also a bit of fear, because I'd never been with someone that close to me who was in the process of dying.

My practice then was very simple: I would just notice all the feelings that were happening in me. For almost a year I would sit, and as I was sitting tears would flow spontaneously, sometimes for an entire hour. But it was a strangely "impartial" experience, because I wasn't participating with it: There wasn't some story. There wasn't any kind of indulgence in the experience, just witnessing this pure grief, and then, quite remarkably, getting up and feeling the day very fresh and lucid.

Anything was permissible on the mat. I didn't have to struggle with or wrestle this experience to the ground, or defend myself from it. I realized then that all those years of practice had made my heart very, very large, had made my mind very, very large, so that they could encompass everything. It was quite remarkable to me that I could have that intense experience of grief and at the same time feel basically content and OK.

Q. *You're describing what some Buddhist traditions call "bare reality," where you meet life "bare and direct" without any story, beyond concepts or commentary.*

A. Very much so. During the first few months after Robert died, I found that there were very few people I could be with who understood. Talk about bare! In those months I felt as though I were being boiled alive. There were other losses as well at that time: I had just lost a partnership of seven years. It was a time of huge loss. The moment I related this grief to many of my friends, they started trying to get rid of it for me. Or they tried to "correct" it, or convince me that it somehow wasn't as bad as it really was. I found this refusal of real experience to be a real act of violence.

I think if I'd gone to my mat feeling that I had to correct myself or make myself better or get rid of this grief, that experience would have been an act of self-refusal and fundamental aggression.

Q. *How has this shaped your understanding of the goal of practice?*

A. I no longer think the unitive state (or enlightenment, if you will) is a place where everything goes swimmingly our way. Or that it's a pie-in-the-sky place where everybody's smiling. When I meet people who proclaim that everything's wonderful, I have an overwhelming desire to go out and buy a handgun. It just doesn't ring true in my direct experience.

Some of the people who have been my teachers, people for whom I have immense regard, have allowed me to see them in the throes of intense struggle and suffering. Yet I know at the same time that they are very much rooted in the ground of their being. This has been an important teaching for me. It shifted my idea of enlightenment. Precisely because they could be so honest with where they were, they expressed a form of enlightenment in their saying, "Hmm, I'm irritable today." That's very enlightened — to be able to admit to one's immediate experience.

Q. *Donna, can you say a little about what is most inspiring to you in your practice these days? What's the cutting edge for you?*

A. Those who know me well won't be surprised at my answer. But my students and people who've read my books might be surprised to know that my primary yoga teachers in the last seven years have had four legs. They're furry. And English. [Laughter!] Horses have truly been my strongest, most powerful yoga teachers in the last seven years. They have made me face things on the mat that probably never would have come up otherwise. They've been my most challenging teachers by far because they've revealed to me deep, hidden levels of violence in myself that I hadn't confronted, levels of impatience that I hadn't seen. Through my deep relationship with horses, I've been faced with confronting the violence that remains within me, toward myself and others.

In a horse you have an animal that is so powerful that it can literally kill you if you're not paying attention — or if you haven't joined with that animal in a spirit of partnership rather than domination or fear-based leadership. If you really haven't joined with that animal in partnership, then your participation with nature is incredibly dangerous.

It's incredibly dangerous even when you have the partnership, but there is some deep, deep, deep level of observation that the horses teach me that wasn't there before. It's a kind of unbounded sensitivity to everything. It makes my hair stand on end when I begin to notice what my horse notices, and then I can see the huge gap in our perceptions. I want to have that unbounded connection with life that my horse has, so I am trying to listen in the way that the animal listens.

Q. *Can you give us an example of what you've learned from your horse?*

A. One day I was riding around a track that my horse and I know very well. We've done it a thousand times. Suddenly he stopped dead in his tracks. I could feel his heart beating a hundred miles an hour and he wasn't going to move. His whole body went rigid. I thought "I can't see a darn thing." I looked and looked and looked and I thought "This is ridiculous." I urged him on. He took a few more steps and went rigid again.

Then I could see what he had noticed: A tree had fallen. There was no way he could really have seen it. He had to have *felt* that that tree had fallen. The trees around it were clearly at risk of falling as well, and I'm sure he could feel that also. I thought: "How distanced we are from the universe that we don't feel those things too — that a tree's fallen." Maybe if I stick around this guru long enough, I will develop that unbounded connection with everything, so that I'll know too when a tree is about to fall or has just fallen.

Q. *It's interesting that you focus on both the beauty and the violent wildness of nature. How does this relate to your yoga practice?*

A. I think this is a paradox of yoga practice: Why don't we seem to integrate practice by becoming chaotic and disorganized and wild and chronically spontaneous? After all, this practice breaks through into our animal nature, doesn't it? The paradox seems to be that through this very ordered, inner tempering we get strong enough, steely enough that we can let go.

There is a metaphor for that in my work with horses. I study horsemanship every day. I go to clinics. It's taken all of that preparation to be able to get on my horse and say, "Go, gallop," and not to hold on. One doesn't start with, "Oh, I'll just get on this horse and go at a flat-out gallop without a saddle or bridle." It might take ten years of training to get to that place. That seems to be the paradox of practice. It takes a simplified, ordered, reliable, ingrained patterning of trust and skillfulness in order to let go, and to ride that level of spiritedness and power within one's life. ●

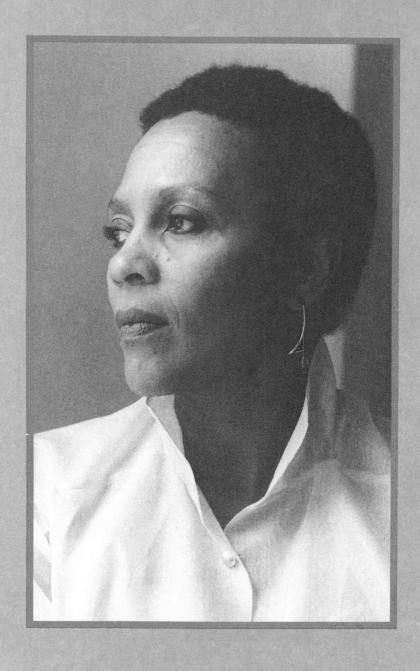

Maya Breuer

FEELING MY WINGS

MAYA BREUER, born Beryl Powers, grew up in Providence, Rhode Island, along with her five siblings. Her family's ancestors hail from a tribe of West African Jews. In high school Maya was interested in philosophy and the arts. Married at age seventeen, Maya is mother to three children, who are all now adults. She attended Rhode Island College, and has worked as an expert in Equal Employment Program Development for the Rhode Island state government, and for various community action programs and Fortune 500 consulting firms and companies. • Maya's life and career took a major turn when she decided to explore her creative self as a visual and jazz artist. She performed extensively throughout the Northeast, appearing in jazz clubs and other venues with notables in the world of jazz. She is considered by many to be one of the finest jazz singers of our time. • After traveling to India to deepen her *sadhana* and study of yoga, Maya incorporated the art of living and teaching yoga into her life. Today she lectures, offers retreats and workshops, trains and certifies others, and remains focused on encouraging and educating minorities to explore the healing benefits of yoga. Maya is now at work on her first book, *Body, Soul, and Spirit: Yoga for Women of Color.* She resides in Warwick, Rhode Island.

" . . . Who comes to a spring thirsty
and sees the moon reflected in it? . . .

Who lets a bucket down and brings up
A flowing prophet? Or like Moses goes for fires
and finds what burns inside the sunrise? . . .

. . . But don't be satisfied with stories, how things
have gone with others. Unfold
your own myth, without complicated explanation,
so everyone will understand the passage
We have opened you."

(From "Unfold Your Own Myth," *The Essential Rumi* translated by
Coleman Barks, HarperSanFrancisco, 1995, page 40-41.)

AS I SIT IN THE LIMOUSINE, my mind has become fixed
on death: the power of death, the silence of death. Today I eulogize
my brother. This is the first of two funerals for him. Tomorrow I will
bring his body home for the final family farewell.

In 1990 my brother died of AIDS. He was in his thirties, and
I was his chief caregiver for more than two and a half years. A graduate of Brown medical school, my brother frowned on my crystals
and yoga practice, but at the end of his life sat with me to do
pranayama. The breathwork helped open him to life as it was passing. Ultimately it opened him to death.

"See now that I, even I, am [God] and there is no [other]
god with me. I kill, and I make alive; I wound, and I heal."
(Deuteronomy 32:39) I remember the songs my great-grandfather
used to sing. Words, breath, tears, and the sting of a life cut short
pour from my being as I speak of this friend, my brother.

In the time before I knew yoga, somehow I lost the beat and breath and ended up alone in a bar with my glass raised, poised to surrender the drink to my lips. The journey of life challenged me on every front. No om. No *shanti*. No Shiva. No *pranayama*. No *pratyahara*. Only mindless, blind existence.

Along the way there were joy-filled moments: the birth of my children, loving relationships. But always the challenges: the loss of a sister to suicide, the untimely death of a mate, life as a nineteen-year-old with three children. Like so many other black women, I found no *sthira sukha* (steadiness or ease), only endless effort. *Duhkha,* the pain and bruises of life, set me up to be a seeker.

With three children, very respectable work, and a busy, productive life, it never occurred to me that I had a drinking problem. But I am a recovering alcoholic. During the time I was taking care of my dying brother, I would frequently need a drink to calm down. One day I was so badly hung over I couldn't get to him to take care of his needs. Later we talked and I began to realize that, yes, I had a drinking problem. The words of a Negro spiritual I learned in childhood came back to me:

> "There must be a God somewhere,
> And he helps me when my load
> gets so very hard to bear.
> And when I rise from dark despair,
> He surmounts my every care,
> And my heart tells me that surely
> There is a God somewhere."

My childhood contained the seeds of my life as a yogini. Born into an extremely religious family, I grew up with the prayers and spirituals of black Orthodox Jews, descendants of a community that originated in Ethiopia in the 1880s. My ancestors were slaves who had chosen to reclaim their ancient roots in Judaism. Thus, I fasted, prayed, listened to the sound of trumpets in homage to the conch, and took in the first dharma lessons from my great-grandfather, a composer, and my grandfather, a singer of these psalms.

Each song in longing or in praise of God helped lay the foundation for my practice. Each was a gift of my connection to spirit. The discipline and structure of my Orthodox Jewish upbringing helped solidify my commitment to *sadhana*.

I came to yoga in 1979 at the First Unitarian Church in Providence, Rhode Island. I was seeking reality. Paramahansa Yogananda was my first teacher. Through his book *Autobiography of a Yogi,* I learned that there might be another way. Next the child yogi, Maharaji, taught me how to meditate. I kissed his feet, though at the same time wondering about the hierarchy, the guru, and my lack of importance in the grand scheme of things.

In 1988 I traveled to Kripalu Center, met Yogi Amrit Desai, and became initiated. Through the practices I received from Amrit, I came to know my real guru and teacher, Swami Kripalu, or Bapuji, "beloved father," as we lovingly call him.

I attended many retreats and intensives at Kripalu. Every so often when *samskaras* were released, I'd be overwhelmed and would slip into nearby Lenox for a drink. However, the more I did my practice, the clearer I was. In time it became easier to choose yoga. Meanwhile, Bapuji was in my dreams and with me in waking life. Later, India, magical, mystical, spiritual, beckoned me. Questions flooded in: Why do we suffer? Who created this system where one human being is higher than another, even in India?

"You asked if yoga and meditation have changed my life. My answer is yes. Yoga changed me and then I changed my life."

I made a pilgrimage to India in 1994 to honor Bapuji's memory and visit all the sites touched by his presence. Along with the questions came the openings: My swim in the Narmada River, watching the peacocks dance, hearing jackals howling at night or the local carpenter playing his flute. Walking to temple at dawn, watching the *arti* lamp circle around the dark presence of the statue. Little did I know when I sat sketching the face of a woman taking care of the temple that it would turn out to be Bapuji's sister. There was the taste of a homecoming in all that was strange and different.

Asanas, prayer, *pranayama* — everything I do now is practice: teaching the rudiments of yoga, singing devotional songs, leading retreats for women of color at Kripalu. My practice these days is organic and indigenous, a part of my everyday life, like rice grow-ing out of a riverbed or the fighting between the Yanomamo tribes. I walk and feel my breath. I speak to a young black woman and explain how yoga will calm her mind and help her to feel stronger and clearer. "Just come to a class," I say. In turn my practice responds to each day. Some days my body performs many asanas and other days just a few; I walk in meditation, keeping my heart open, my *citta* aware, my ego quiet, and my feet firmly planted.

You asked if yoga and meditation have changed my life. My answer is yes. Yoga changed me and then I changed my life. Nowadays there is nowhere to go in this moment but in, so I mine and plumb the depths of my being with yoga and meditation. Life continues on life's terms, but I am armed for victory *(ujjayi)!*

I did not come to yoga to stretch. I came to live. ●

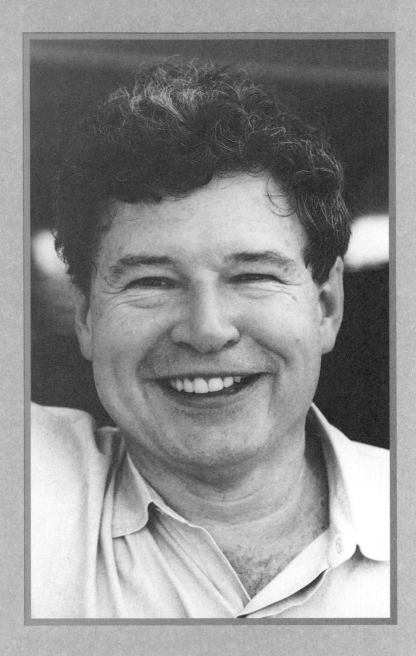

Phillip Moffitt

IT'S NOT PERSONAL!

PHILLIP MOFFITT is the former editor in chief of *Esquire*. At age forty, he abandoned the publishing world to devote himself full time to pursuing the inner life. He began studying *raja* yoga in the Sivananda lineage in the early 1970s and later studied intensively in the Iyengar tradition. Phillip began studying Buddhist meditation in the practice of the Southeast Asian forest tradition, often called "the tradition of the elders," in 1983. He maintains an integrated practice from both the Buddhist and Patanjali traditions. • Phillip teaches Buddhist meditation at retreat centers throughout the United States and also teaches a form of yoga called Mindful Movement™, designed to enhance the meditation experience. He writes the Dharma Wisdom column for *Yoga Journal*, and has a weekly meditation group in San Rafael, California, which is open to all. In 1994 he formed Life Balance Institute, offering programs for aligning your life with your values, regardless of whether you have a spiritual practice. • Phillip is a member of the Teachers' Council at Spirit Rock Meditation Center and is the coauthor of *The Power to Heal* and *Medicine's Great Journey*. He has served on the board of directors of the C. G. Jung Foundation in New York City and on the C. G. Jung Institute Board in San Francisco, and has mentored leaders of nonprofit organizations.

Q. *Has meditation changed your life, Phillip?*

A. The most profound change I'm aware of just now is a growing realization that life is not personal. This may seem a surprising or even strange view to those unfamiliar with Eastern spirituality, but it has powerful implications. It's very freeing to see that events in my life are arising because of circumstances in which I'm involved, but that I'm not at the *center* of them in any particular way. They're impersonal. They're arising because of causes and conditions. They are not "me." There is a profound freedom in this. It makes life much more peaceful and harmonious because I'm not in reaction to events all the time.

When I began to realize this — not as a philosophy from an ancient text, but rather as my own direct experience — it changed my life. Having this direct experience of the impersonal nature of life allows me not to get caught, not to take everything so personally. Therefore I'm much more likely to be able to maintain the intention of which the Buddha speaks: I can reflect my true values. Rather than saying, for example, "How dare you say that to me," or "I won't put up with that" — making a particular situation into a big drama — I can relax around it. This way of being leads to a much greater sense of ease in the world. Life is difficult by definition, but this shift makes it all profoundly easier.

I see my students' lives also being changed by this insight. My students have always been some of my best teachers. Over the last couple of years, I've been working with a student who's had a series of emotional and environmental challenges in his life. I see the way in which this understanding of the impersonal nature of life has radically transformed him. It's taken two years of repeating this view to him over and over, but just this one understanding has changed how much actual physical suffering there is for him. As he has learned in his yoga not to take the body's reaction *personally,* he's discovered that there is no "me" or "my" in the center of his experience, just a series of chemical reactions because of causes and circumstances. As a result there is no longer the added chemical reaction of fear and aversion to the pain. He can relate more directly to the *pain itself.*

With this new view, he doesn't have to spin into additional suffering. His body's reactions are dramatically softened, and the change in the internal, emotional experience of his mind is like night to day. This is one of the central insights of the contemplative traditions: The difference between pain and that same pain multiplied by resistance to the pain is enormous. Science supports this. It's not a speculative philosophy. And, of course, the wonderful thing is that this all applies to our lives as they are right now, not at some future time "when I become a great yogi" or get to some future enlightened place.

I believe that one of the most transformative things we learn in any kind of mindfulness meditation is precisely this kind of tolerance: being able to stay present with experience without contracting into it. Contracting into something is to take it extremely personally.

The Buddhist teacher Ajahn Sumedho has greatly influenced my ability to be with things the way they are. He stresses the Buddhist view of the "suchness of things" so beautifully. He says over and over again "This moment is like this." Your knee is hurting? Ah, "Knee pain is like this." Oh, my feelings just got hurt. "Hurt feelings are like this." When you say "This moment is like this," you are depersonalizing it. It doesn't mean you're giving up your relationship to it. In fact, if you don't take it all so personally, you actually have a wider range of possibilities of responding to any and all moments in your life.

With this skill, life gets richer, not less rich, which is one of those paradoxes about the Eastern approach. Often people say, "Oh yeah, but meditation deadens you to life. Who wants to have that kind of boring life?" It's not that way at all. In fact, you have your full range of responses available to you because you're not caught in your contraction, your aversion, or your preconceived ideas about how it should be. Not at all. You get to see just "how it is."

Q. *What are your primary practices these days?*

A. In 1983 I began studying Vipassana meditation. I've been a committed practitioner ever since. I've also been a longtime student of yoga. These two traditions — yoga and Buddhism — have an enormous amount in common, of course, and even today I continue to have teachers from both Hindu lineages and Buddhist lineages. The teachings of Patanjali and the Buddha are more similar, I think, than most people realize.

In any event, it's been important for me to continue to study within both traditions, just as a number of teachers in the Buddhist world study with teachers from various Buddhist lineages. This ecumenical approach has been a fact of life throughout the history of Buddhism, and I deeply hope that it's one of the things that continue in the West.

These days my primary practice is meditation. Almost every day I do a *metta,* or lovingkindness, practice that varies in length. I've probably not missed four days of *metta* in five years. I also do Vipassana almost every day. Then, depending on all sorts of things, I either do a formal hatha yoga practice or some other practice as many days in the week as I can. Mostly, though, I am concentrated on actually living the dharma. I try to make each moment of my life a moment of practice rather than have practice be something that I go off to do.

It's interesting for me to look back on the way my *metta* practice evolved. I was a person who had natural ease with *samadhi* practice. I had wonderful bliss states with *samadhi,* so when I first encountered Vipassana and was asked to give up those delightful altered states, it was difficult.

Then another surrender was required. No sooner had I started opening to Vipassana — the practice of choiceless awareness where there is no one object but you open to whatever is arising — than my teacher introduced to me the idea of *metta* meditation. Another practice??!! I was very resistant, to say the least. I thought *metta* practice was sentimental. It seemed to be trying to promote a kind of happiness that sounded, well, artificial.

My first response was simply not to go into the hall when *metta* was being practiced. When *metta* started I would just leave. After a few days of getting more and more uncomfortable with myself over that, I thought, "Well, if I'm going to have such a strong negative opinion about this practice that is 'breaking up the wonderful Vipassana work,' at least I ought to go see what it is."

It was a great moment when I said that. I went in and the experience of the *metta* practice was deep and rich. If you tell someone about *metta* practice, it can seem hokey, but the actual experience is really wonderful because you're engaging the heart in basic relatedness to life.

In our modern time what's rewarded in our society is not so much a *relatedness* to life but a *manipulation* of life. There's selling people things, there's trying to get to the top of the ladder and out-do, and competition, competition, competition. There's very little time for developing relatedness in our everyday life. In practice communities a great deal of time is spent in a kind of relatedness activity, which creates a bond of community and a sense of caring. It is not personalized in a sense, it is just related. The *metta* has a very positive effect in that regard.

Metta is also helpful in keeping us from getting too rigid in practice situations. There is a kind of determination in deep practice that involves a certain discipline, and there's a tendency for people to think that discipline is rigid. It can look rigid, but at the center of it there's a softening, a surrendering of the heart. *Metta* helps keep our heart in that softened place.

In my experience, all meditation practice is a surrendering more than an achieving, because if you try to make it too much achieving, you end up in duality again. There's a feeling of "There is something I'm not that I must be," which creates two selves. There is this self *now* and there is this *future* self, both of which are going to suffer. But if one surrenders to the inherent wisdom of the mind, one discovers that it's all already moving in the right direction.

"You just stay in the moment; stay with the sensations just as they are; stay with it *just as it is*. This is the path."

As one surrenders to this inherent wisdom, one develops what's called in Buddhism "clear comprehension." One knows what is appropriate action, right action. Again, coming full circle, this right action is not personal. These actions don't come from a clinging to "me" or "mine," but directly from clear comprehension.

This is action that does not come out of reaction — either craving or aversion. What's pleasant will arrive and what's unpleasant will arrive, naturally. Those things don't go away; they are inherent in the moment. That's *vedana,* or feeling, the second foundation of Mindfulness. It's inherent: it arises with the moment.

Real freedom, however, is precisely not being identified with *vedana* in a way that causes you to act unskillfully. You don't identify with the feelings of pleasant or unpleasant because you come to see that identification with them is a misperception. It's not that you are getting rid of something when you stop the identification; you're just clarifying a misperception.

Q. *So this lack of identification is a fruit that comes from practice?*

A. Exactly! You don't quite acquire it, you just do the practice, see clearly, and then you get the fruit because you've seen clearly. You don't have to go reach for the fruit. You just stay in the practice. You just stay in the moment; stay with the sensations just as they are; stay with it *just as it is*. This is the path.

It's a wonderful way to live, because it allows you to be with this very moment. And this very moment is where the life is. You don't have to be a meditator or a yoga practitioner for this to be true. It's true for every living being: This moment is where the life is.

Learning to come into this moment as it is with our inherent values — lovingkindness and compassion and the desire not to do harm — is the way to come into life, no matter what your religious beliefs are. We're not talking about a belief system; we're talking about living life — for all beings. Paradoxically, when we can let it not be about "me" and "mine," we are free to let more and more of life flow through us without contracting, closing down, holding on, or pushing away. It's an easier way to live in the world. It's a way that's full of life. ●

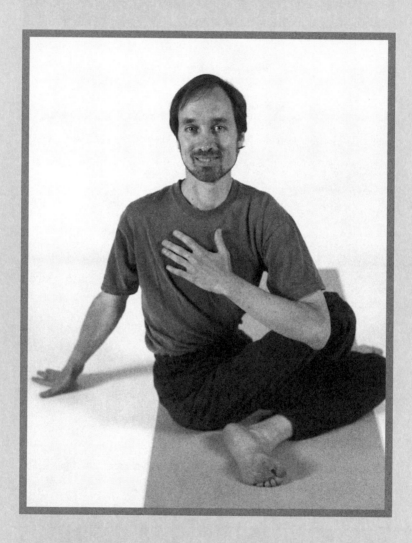

Richard Faulds

PRACTICE, PRACTICE, PRACTICE

RICHARD FAULDS embarked on the spiritual path through a defining moment in Little League baseball that led him to believe in himself. Known at Kripalu by his Sanskrit name, Shobhan, he began a self-taught yoga practice in his teens and started meditating during his undergraduate years at Vanderbilt University. Profoundly at a loss for how to make his way in the world, Shobhan earned his law degree from the Dickinson School of Law while dreaming of being an organic farmer with sufficient free time to practice yoga. While a law student, Shobhan met his much-loved wife, Danna, and they embarked headlong on the Kripalu path of transformation. A Legal Aid attorney before moving into the Kripalu community, Shobhan was the ashram's legal counsel for a decade. • After leaving Kripalu, he completed a master's program in counseling and human development at Radford University, which integrated East and West for him. Shobhan returned to Kripalu in 1998 to serve as president for three years. He currently chairs Kripalu's board of trustees and is the author of *Kripalu Yoga: A Guide to Practice On and Off the Mat*. • Shobhan and Danna live in the Shenandoah Valley of Virginia, where they practice yoga, tend a large vegetable garden, and host individuals and small groups interested in practicing and passing on the teachings of the Kripalu tradition.

IN THE SPRING OF 1981 I strode across the stage to receive my college diploma and proceeded directly to Kripalu Yoga Ashram, a young man on a spiritual quest. Much to my parents' dismay, the impact of four years of academic study on my developing psyche paled in comparison to my forays into the burgeoning world of American spirituality. Something in me was waking up, and I was inexorably drawn to anything that promised to expand my horizons. I scanned bulletin boards for workshop flyers, joined meditation groups, and visited communes. My backpack always sported a paperback or library volume on some unconventional topic.

More than anything, I was fascinated by the teachings and techniques of yoga. I learned the basic yoga postures, mostly from books, and did them daily. After two years of steady practice, I sensed their transformative power and wanted to go deeper. Winding down the gravel road to the rural retreat, I wondered what it would be like to meet a yoga master in the flesh.

No amount of practice could have prepared me for that encounter. As the sixty-eight-year-old Swami Kripalu walked into the room, my mind was catapulted into a state of focused awareness deeper than anything I had ever experienced. My first startled thought was that he looked surprisingly like my grandfather, who was also bald and pencil thin. But the similarities ended there. Swami Kripalu was a lightning bolt wrapped in an orange linen robe. The energy that emanated from him was palpable, an amalgamation of intimate love and sheer spiritual power. His facial expressions and gestures were mesmerizing to watch, shifting back and forth between childlike playfulness and stern truth-telling, enabling him to communicate with the hundred or so people gathered there without saying a word.

A chant started and the room became drunk on his energy. Most people became giddy with laughter and danced with joyous abandon. Some sobbed quietly. A few fell into trance and lost all outward consciousness. It was clear to me that Swami Kripalu was not doing anything to make all this happen. Somehow he had purified his body, mind, and heart in a way that allowed the full force of his being to flow through him. The result was mind-boggling.

Before Swami Kripalu entered that room, I felt pretty good about myself as a spiritual seeker. As he walked out, I was plunged into a deep existential crisis. Swami Kripalu's purity was like a spotlight shining on my artifice. His depth and clarity made my superficiality and confusion stand out in bold relief. Seeing so clearly what is possible through yoga, I felt profoundly inadequate. Convinced there was no pathway leading from where I was to where I felt called to go, I returned home in a hopeless state. Desperate for guidance, I began to read Swami Kripalu's writings, searching for some clue on how to proceed down the spiritual path. What I found was a call to practice as reflected in the following excerpts from his writing:

> To read uplifting books or listen to spiritual discourses is good. But to practice even a little is of the utmost importance. The profound meaning of yoga is

understood only by those who study it systematically through personal practice. The day you start to practice, your true progress will begin.

Accepting the truth proclaimed by the scriptures does not produce knowledge. Real knowledge is only obtained through direct experience. For experience, practice is indispensable. Knowledge without experience is false knowledge.

Through various yoga experiences, a seeker goes on intensifying his faith, courage, knowledge, zeal, and devotion. In this way he progresses on the path of yoga, gaining the knowledge of yoga through the practice of yoga.

I learned that Swami Kripalu had lived in seclusion for thirty years, spending ten hours a day in meditation and intensive yoga practice. He encouraged householders to live a loving, truthful, and healthy lifestyle, practicing as much as their family circumstances allowed. If only fifteen minutes were available morning and night, they should be spent in devotional activities such as prayer, mantra repetition, chanting the name of the Lord, and heartfelt worship. If an hour a day were available, yoga or sitting meditation could be practiced. Those wanting to make substantial spiritual progress were encouraged to devote at least two hours to yoga, breathing exercises, and meditation. The purpose of practice was to learn how to drop beneath the choppy surface of awareness, and dive deeply into the ocean of intelligent energy that is the spiritual source of body and mind.

> "By bringing me back again and again to the felt sense of my body and the steady flow of breath, practice began to peel away the layers of tension, repression, and denial that were sustaining my sorry state of affairs."

My depression lifted and a firm determination arose within me. Regardless of my shortcomings, I could practice. An hour of yoga was already a part of my morning routine. I got up earlier to add an hour of meditation, using a technique taught by Swami Kripalu. Morning after morning I nurtured my body, allowing energy to flow and awareness to sink deep within. Day after day I aspired to live from a place of energetic connection. I continued this practice throughout graduate school, cultivating relationships with others living this Kripalu lifestyle. I joined the resident staff of Kripalu Center, a vibrant community founded in part on the maxim "Practice, practice, practice." When I eventually left the resident community, practice became the cornerstone on which I built an independent life. After all these years it is only fitting to ask: "What has practice brought me?"

My initial years of practice were a time of internal struggle and healing. Somewhere in the process of growing into adulthood, I had lost touch with the essential me. At first I was just aware that deep down something was missing. Eventually I came to see that this vague sense of malaise was a symptom of a much larger problem: The flow of energy through my being was blocked on every level. Some parts of my body were chronically tense and others almost numb. Relationships and incidents from my past were unresolved, and I actively resisted feelings of anger and sadness that tried to surface in my awareness. Rigid belief systems filtered and obscured my view of reality, leading me to blame the world for my troubles and see myself as either unsung hero or helpless victim.

By bringing me back again and again to the felt sense of my body and the steady flow of breath, practice began to peel away the layers of tension, repression, and denial that were sustaining my sorry state of affairs. Kripalu yoga's emphasis on self-acceptance played a critical role in my safe passage through this stage of practice. Adopting the inner attitude that Swami Kripalu called "self-observation without judgment" helped me begin to hear the powerful voices of fear and self-judgment that lay beneath many of my unconscious patterns.

As greater self-awareness dawned, my practice shifted from what yoga calls *purification* to what psychology calls *growth*. Yoga and meditation became a way to remain intimate with my inner experience despite the bumps and bruises of life. Practice served as a safe haven where the waters of life flowed freely and the lamp of awareness burned more or less brightly. I spent time there daily to recharge, let off steam, and recalibrate my mind.

Off the mat, life's challenges were presenting me with innumerable opportunities to apply what I had learned through yoga and meditation. In the midst of a busy professional life, it took everything I could muster to stay grounded in my body, remain relaxed in the face of fear, and respond directly to whatever was happening in the present moment. My inner and outer worlds, once entirely separate, were coming together. Where I had struggled to keep my head above water, practice was teaching me how to swim in the river of life.

> "Instead of pole-vaulting me over the troubles of life, practice makes possible the strength of character and steadiness of mind to fully experience whatever life brings."

At times life is a ruthless teacher, purifying the body despite discomfort, stripping away mental masks and defenses despite fear. Two years ago I was diagnosed with a rare type of benign tumor that destroyed my right ankle joint. Two surgeries and an artificial ankle later, I am still not back on my feet. For quite a while during this time, practice was a raw experience. Yoga was a daily confrontation with my limitations, letting go of all the standing postures and other exercises I could no longer do. Meditation was watching the cherished dream that my wife and I would climb mountains into our nineties dissolve before my eyes. At times like these, practice becomes simply bearing the truth.

On an external level, my condition torpedoed the vigorous life I knew and loved. But each morning, practice helps me see that on a more fundamental level, nothing has changed. I still wake up to the same choices: Am I going to be happy today? Am I going to face the day's challenges directly and honestly? Am I going to live in accord with the truth that all is well? Beyond that, I have to admit that this difficult experience has brought me very real benefits. I appreciate life's wonderful moments more and sweat the small stuff less. Where before I made my way through airports and shopping malls blind to such things, I now notice people everywhere on crutches and in wheelchairs, usually dealing with far worse maladies than mine. Having had to contend with my own limitations, I am far more patient and understanding of others.

One might ask: "Are these the benefits of practice or the result of a significant health challenge?" I can say without hesitation that there was every opportunity to harden against the perceived unfairness of my plight. It would have been easy to poison my life, and the lives of those around me, and rationally justify it. Only the grace born of practice allowed me to choose differently. No matter how painful, I know that reality is a better place to hang my hat than self-deception. Slowly the realization has come that practice is not a way to dodge the pain inherent in life and death. On the contrary, practice is a collision course with everything that stands between me and the way things are. Instead of pole-vaulting me over the troubles of life, practice makes possible the strength of character and steadiness of mind to fully experience whatever life brings. All that said, I hope to walk normally again, preferably sooner than later!

> "The end result is this: In the midst of a messy human life, I often feel whole and complete."

What inspires me to keep practicing? Practice calls forth the best of me, invoking a relaxed state of being that is both self-fulfilling and a powerful catalyst for growth and transformation. As I sit down to meditate, the process of going inside begins. Breath flows. Feelings clear. Thoughts settle. Challenges and issues resolve so predictably that I keep a notepad nearby my cushion to jot down solutions, allowing me to forget problems entirely. On most days absorption comes easily and the barrier between inside and outside falls away. I have found no pleasure that compares with the joy of effortless being.

The essence of my current practice is simplicity itself: I use the techniques of yoga to embrace what is. I don't strive to make anything happen. I don't suppress anything that wants to happen. I allow life to be. Moments of exaltation, a devotional sense of communion with Spirit, and a strong pull toward mystical union are not strangers to me. While I am not "established in my true nature" as described in the scriptures, I know that the enlightened state is the very ground of my being, the natural state of everyone and everything, a perpetually open door to walk through anytime. The end result is this: In the midst of a messy human life, I often feel whole and complete.

A few months after that first visit to Kripalu Yoga Ashram, I called back to see when Swami Kripalu would appear again in public. I was shocked to learn that he had returned to India and died within a matter of weeks. Although it could be said that my single meeting with him established the trajectory of my life, I think Swami Kripalu would say that he just introduced me to practice. Practice accomplished all the rest. ●

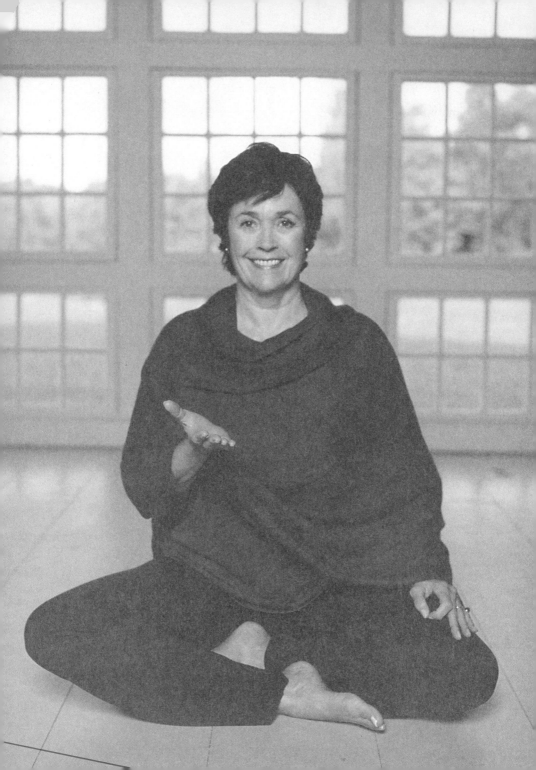

Lilias Folan

CULTIVATING WITNESS CONSCIOUSNESS

LILIAS FOLAN is the host of the groundbreaking PBS-TV series *Lilias, Yoga and You!* which was nationally syndicated to 260 PBS stations from 1970 to 1985. She later created a 52-part hatha yoga series entitled *Lilias!* which aired on PBS from 1978 to 1996. *Time* magazine has called Lilias "the Julia Child of Yoga." • Lilias attended Bennington College, where she studied painting, drawing, and the Italian language. She began her practice of yoga in 1964, studying with Swami Vishnu Devananda of the Sivananda lineage. In 1973 she traveled to India to study Vedanta philosophy and meditation under the tutelage of Swami Chidananda of the Divine Light Society in Rishikesh. She continued her meditation practice with Swami Muktananda. • Lilias's hatha practice and teaching has been deeply influenced by T. K. V. Desikachar, Angela Farmer, and B. K. S. Iyengar. In 1998, Goswami Kriyananda of the Temple of Kyriya Yoga Seminary bestowed upon her the title of Swami Kavitananda, "one who knows bliss through motion and poetry." • Lilias is the author of *Lilias Yoga and You, Yoga and Your Life*, and *Lilias! Yoga Gets Better with Age*. She has also hosted many hatha yoga videos for home practice. Lilias resides in Cincinnati, Ohio.

Q. Lilias, I'm imagining that because of the longevity of your TV program, you've taught yoga to more people in the world than any other teacher ever has — living or dead!

A. I think you may be right. Possibly millions of students — all ages, sizes, and shapes — began their yoga practice with me on PBS. And the program still airs in different parts of the country, believe it or not!

Q. In many ways your televised classes have been a wonderful bridge into yoga for a cross section of Americans who might never otherwise have found their way to the mat. How did the TV program originate?

A. *Lilias, Yoga and You!* came on the air in 1972, originating right here in the Midwest, at WCET, Cincinnati, Ohio. Within months it was airing nationally on PBS.

Q. How do you account for the meteoric rise of the TV show so early in the development of interest in yoga in this country?

A. I think I was just in the right place at the right time — doing what I was supposed to be doing. Bob — my wonderful husband of many years — and I were living in New York City when we discovered that he needed to move to Cincinnati for his work. This was in the late 1960s. We were trying to move, but my house just wasn't selling. So I did what any good yoga person would do — I went to a psychic to find out when the house would find a buyer!

The psychic was a wonderful woman in New York City named Beulah Brown. To make a long story short, I wrote out a question for her, which she then picked out of a wicker basket. The question, of course, was, "When will my house sell?" She said, "You will sell your house when the tulips bloom. But stand up! Stand up! I have another message for you. I see cameras and lights around you and you'd better be ready." That was two years before the television show really exploded on PBS.

Q. *Lilias, you've been practicing yoga for well over thirty years, and you've often told me that your practice has stayed very fresh. What's the cutting edge of your practice right now?*

A. I think it's listening to my heart and everything that that means. I think we grow into the experiences that we have that are mystical. It's taken me thirty, maybe forty years to understand certain experiences I had in my early years. I had a few powerful experiences of a spiritual nature. But I didn't understand them earlier in my life. Actually, I didn't understand myself then either. I always felt that I wasn't really good enough. I looked around and thought everyone else was having these fabulous lives and experiences, and I wasn't. Getting to know myself has been the core of my continual journey in yoga. I've come to trust that we all have what I would call a "spiritual heart," a capacity for profound love, and a capacity for knowing God.

Karen Armstrong wrote a fascinating book called *A History of God*. She said something that really caught my attention: In primitive times everyone had a — I think she used the word "God-hole." Everyone had a place in them that was connected to the divine. As the centuries have rolled by, that connection, that God space, has grown a kind of membrane over it. Many of us who have come back and are in this life now have felt the longing for that God-hole to be filled again. Now I understand that that's what I've been longing for. For so many years I looked for that love in all the wrong places, not understanding that it was really about reconnecting to the divine Light within.

Q. *Can you say something about where you had been looking for it?*

A. Well, I always thought it was going to be out there — in the monastery, ashram, or convent. In somebody else. Or in some thing I could get that was outside me. It took me so long to understand that it's inside, to understand that it has many ingredients to it — ingredients like thankfulness and gratitude and celebration and lovingkindness. These ineffable qualities describe what's going on inside the Heart.

Q. *How did this discovery enter into your teaching of yoga?*

A. I know that everyone has this same longing. I know that everyone can reconnect with her heart. The first thing I have students do is to ask themselves, "Where do you feel love in your body?" I ask them to close their eyes and put their hand there. Well, everyone, young and old, puts their hands on their chest. Then I ask them to please open their eyes and notice that no one has put their hand on their big toe.

Heart feelings do not come from the bottoms of your feet. They come from the center of your chest. It is about feeling. It is not about thinking, though I've come to understand that the heart does think. But it's not the kind of thought that comes from my brain. The heart has its own intelligence. Learning and accepting that has been an important part of the path for me. For me, recognizing the true source of this love has been the central aspect of my realization in yoga.

Q. *Do you view your success and fame differently as a result of this realization?*

A. Well, it's so short-lived — the new house and new car, a new swimming pool. The thrill of it is so short-lived — like a new lover, a new dress. The euphoria is very short-lived and then you're right back where you started. The truth of the matter is this kind of God-love is a constant flow and there's plenty for everyone. There's plenty for everyone. I remember thinking with my firstborn, how could I love anything more than this son. And then a second son arrived and, looking into his eyes, I realized there was plenty of love for everyone.

Q. *You've talked about the emptiness of external things, and coming to understand that those things are finally very disappointing — not our true source. I wonder if you're an example of somebody who's come to understand the emptiness of external objects through actually having plenty of them. Some people come to disappointment through failure in the externals —*

through not getting what they want. Perhaps you have come to this kind of disappointment through getting it. Is that fair?

A. Very much so. It's a little scary, but I think I have learned the meaning of Christ's parable of walking on the water. The trick is to take one step at a time and not look down. Just as you've said, there has been affluence and looking for love in all the wrong places and fame. As soon as you look down at all that, you begin evaluating and thinking you're "hot stuff." That makes you sink down into it all — drowning in all the thickness. You've got to come back up and continue on, one step as a time. I've found this a peaceful and interesting practice: Grace keeps rolling the ocean in front of my feet, sort of like a magic carpet, in the moment, one step at a time.

Q. *I believe the Buddha once said, "Fame is the deadliest poison." Yet you seem to have thrived on it. What have been the most positive aspects of your fame?*

A. Well, I don't think I'm really famous, but I'm grateful to have so many friends in the yoga community. I love people. I truly do. I love meeting my "unseen class" out there behind the camera over all these years. I love meeting people heart to heart, and face-to-face. When people say thank you to me, I stop and allow myself to absorb it and then let the compliment flow on through. These have been the parts that I have really savored: giving and receiving love. But thinking you're special or famous can be a deadly poison. The Buddha was absolutely right. We see examples all around us.

Q. *How has your asana practice been part of your spiritual maturing?*

A. There is no question that practicing asanas helped to awaken spontaneously in me what we call in yoga "the witness." Witness consciousness. At first this process happened almost without my awareness. I was stretching, concentrating, focusing inward, and I began to develop the rudiments of this inner seer. No one was saying to me, "Lilias, this is what you should be developing." It was just happening quite naturally.

Practicing asanas began to teach me about myself. They became what Jean Klein used to call one's "closest natural environment." The body is such a great school of learning. It makes you pay attention. I started from the physical part and later began to get the mental benefits. It was a huge day when I actually began to see that I am *not* my thoughts. What a relief! This is *sakshin,* the witness self. It was a real milestone in my practice. Actually it was quite a shock to see what I was thinking and the content of it, the blah-blah of it. The mind just carrying on. Blah, blah, blah!!

Q. *What have been the deepest sources of your inspiration, Lilias?*

A. I had awfully good guidance in my early years. Swami Chidananda, of the Divine Life Society, came to New York in the late '60s. It was like meeting St. Francis of Assisi. It was such a blessing to me to have him take the torch full of fire and light my heart. He said to me, "Get on with it." What he meant by that was "You've got a short life here and it's such a gift to have life. Don't fritter it away. Be up and doing — know yourself as divine and serve." The service part is central to it all.

That was my foundation. It was an authenic yoga foundation — straight from Rishikesh, India, from the real McCoy. First, of course, I studied with Swamiji in New York. Then I went to India — I think I had my thirty-fifth birthday in India with him. I spent a lot of time with him. He came to our home here in America and stayed with us two or three times. It made a huge difference in my family. He is like part of my family: They all know and adore him.

Swamiji is my root teacher. He awakened my heart and is always with me. But the gurus that inspire me day in and day out are my family: my sons and grandchildren, my husband and my daughters-in-law, and our relationships together. What it pulls out of me! The best teaching is right here in the family. I didn't have to go to an ashram to find truth, wisdom, clarity, and humility; I find it very much within my family. It hasn't been all roses. It's been very challenging. I meet all sides of myself coming and going, the positive and the negative. My family push buttons I never knew I had!

Q. *We're all looking for role models as we think about aging. You're doing it so gracefully. What kind of shifts have you noticed in your practice as you moved into your sixties?*

A. Actually I'm in my late sixties now and I'm looking at my life with great appreciation that today is here. Many people don't get to sixty-seven years old. Yes, my practice has changed over the years, and I've had to make some adaptations to aging. At this stage of practice, the asanas have become wonderfully meditative and focused. I'm listening to my body and giving it what it needs each day, and I hope I can keep enthusiastic about the practice.

I teach so very much that I've found that staying inspired is extremely important. Always learning. Taking other teachers' classes. Finding new aspects of the practice. What I feel renewed excitement about right now is my breathing *(pranayama)* practice. Richard Rosen's book, *The Yoga of Breath: A Step-by-Step Guide to Pranayama,* has really inspired me. It's so much more than a breathing book. It's spiritually enlightening.

Q. *What kinds of challenges do you encounter in practice now?*

A. Well, I do have moments of occasional depression. It will sort of roll in. I'm not so afraid of it anymore. I'm not so afraid of fear. I'm much more willing to sit and welcome the fear, the sadness, the depression, to sit in my lap for a little while, and that's OK. My attitude now is "Let's just hang here for a while with this." I ask myself — and listen very carefully — "What are you feeling with the fear?" Old memories still come up, of course. And I say, "OK, don't push them down, Lilias. Bring them into your lap for a little bit."

I have different techniques to not push down my experience and not spiritualize it to death. I have certain ways to address it, feel it, and just lift it up, lift it up into the flame and let it go.

Q. *A lot of Americans are under the misapprehension that by the time you're fifty or so, you should have all your stuff worked out with your parents and your childhood. It's just not like that, is it, Lilias?*

A. It is really not like that. It is amazing to see what comes up these days. And the witness just watches, and stays present, and goes, "Wow." You know the expression "What the mind has long forgotten, the body remembers." There you are in the midst of a yoga asana and up comes the old embarrassing or hurtful picture of something that happened when you were ten. The practice is to stop, look, and listen. Stop and look at it, and listen and feel it. Sometimes I can laugh about it all. I have a mantra sometimes: All it is is "shhhhhhhhh." "Shhhh" quiets the electrical impulses in my brain and allows me just to relax, exhale, and let it go.

Q. *I think there's a way in which practice matures us so we can actually bear seeing those difficult things, don't you?*

A. That's why I like being in my sixties now, because I feel stronger and more able to forgive myself and others. I'm not as vulnerable, and I'm less armored. I'm really, really willing to do this kind of inner work because I know the powerful results. The results are so plain: There's healing and forgiveness and deeper understanding. Let's not forget to laugh at our humanity, our foibles. I find that there is more perspective now. It's a great relief to be free. The witness is alive and well, one step, one moment at a time. Yoga works! •

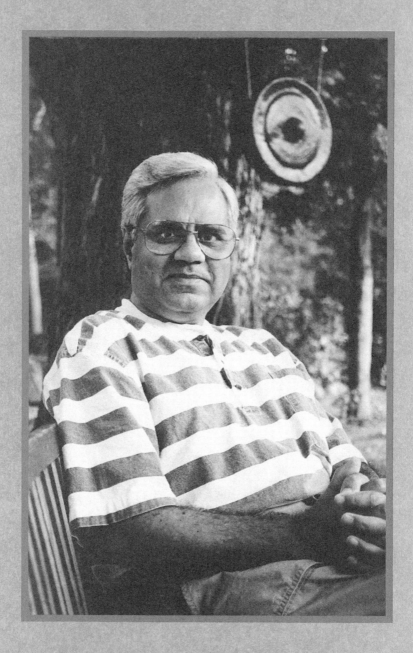

Mu Soeng

LETTING THINGS UNFOLD

Born in India, **MU SOENG** finds a home in the Sino-Korean Buddhist tradition as well as postmodern deconstructionist philosophy. He was a Zen monk for twelve years, and is currently the director of Barre Center for Buddhist Studies, where he helps support the integration of Buddhist contemplative practices with its vigorous scholarly tradition. • Mu Soeng's primary commitment is to the mind with which the Buddha sat under the Bodhi tree prior to his enlightenment experience rather than to codified teachings, yet is an honoring of the codified teachings that provide the framework for personal and societal ethics essential to an optimal functioning in the world. He is the author of *Thousand Peaks: Korean Zen — Tradition and Teachers; Heart Sutra: Ancient Buddhist Wisdom in the Light of Quantum Reality;* and *The Diamond Sutra: Transforming the Way We Perceive the World.* He is working on a commentary on the poem by the Third Ancestor of Zen.

I FIRST BECAME INTERESTED IN ZEN BUDDHISM as a result of a fair amount of reading in existentialist literature. My thinking and orientation have always been socialist, and the basic premises of existentialism seemed to fit very nicely into my personal and societal concerns. A concurrent, albeit accidental, reading of Carlos Castaneda's books in the early '70s seemed to invite an engagement with a direct experience of things.

The very first time I sat a meditation retreat in a formal Zen setting, I had a remarkable direct experience: During the first two thirty-minute sittings, there were periods when my consciousness seemed to transcend time and space. I experienced a "peace that passeth understanding." That first experience has always been a foundational text for me. It is something that I know is possible as direct experience for anyone regardless of who they are and how they think about things. I was fortunate to have that first experience of personal peace, and even more fortunate to find an environment in which to cultivate that peace as a long-term orientation.

The fruit that came out of my first profound experience was that the "teachings" became so much easier to listen to and integrate, without putting up any resistance. It did help perhaps that I was born in India and shared the world-view of the First Noble Truth of the Buddha: Our human condition is characterized by suffering, or *dukkha*. What that first experience showed me was that *dukkha,* the unsatisfactoriness of existence, was self-made, created by my own thinking. Part of that fruit was also a faith or trust in the teachings, in not a scriptural but an existential sense.

The unfolding of my personal practice since that time has been a seamless integration of experience and the truth spoken by the Buddhist traditions about that experience. An aspect of the integration has been to live more and more in the "not knowing" dimension that the Zen tradition talks about. Simply put, this "not knowing" means not trying to force anything — letting things unfold in their own way. There is a deep trust that everything is a karmic process and needs to unfold according to karmic causes and conditions. This is by no means a passive stance but rather an ever-present reminder of the consequence of "leaning into things."

Dogen Zenji said, "To carry yourself forward and experience myriad things is delusion. To know that myriad things come forth and experience themselves is awakening." The maturity of practice for me has been to continue to ground myself in the insight/teaching that the world of samsara is composed of empty phenomena rolling on. Things come into being because of personal and collective karma. There's no abiding core to be found underneath all these karmic formations.

In the face of the empty phenomena, the only thing one can do as "practice" is to not take any ideological position that privileges one thing over another. At the same time, one functions in the world through *upaya,* or "skillful means" — making choices that are not harmful to oneself or others. I am always a bit wary of the transition to "helping others," even though that is a bedrock principle of the Mahayana *bodhisattva* model. The transition can be made, but it needs to be done very carefully, making sure that it's not coming out of any residue of self-deception.

The basic template of the eightfold path of Buddha, triangulated into *sila* (living), *samadhi* (direct personal experience), and *prajna* (nonverbal, nonintellectual understanding), has progressively become the core inspiration for me over the years. I find that in order for practice to mature, there has to be a perfect balance among these three aspects of our existential being (yes, the issue is still existential, not metaphysical).

> " 'Not knowing' means not trying to force anything — letting things unfold in their own way. There is a deep trust that everything is a karmic process and needs to unfold according to karmic causes and conditions."

Another core inspiration comes from case #12 of the koan collection called *Wu-men-kwan,* or Gateless Gate, about "not deceiving yourself." The issue of delusion and awakening, I believe, is a matter of life and death, and not deceiving myself is a subtle, endless process integral to any waking up that might take place. We deceive ourselves when we "lean into things," and part of my own cultivation has been not to lean into things — in other words, to stay away from the most subtle and deceptive forms of self-aggrandizement. That's not an easy job in this very complex society.

> " 'The more you talk and think about it, the further astray you wander from the truth. Stop talking and thinking, and there is nothing you will not be able to know.' "

What keeps coming back again and again as core inspiration for me is the teaching of the now-streaming "this moment" in which "nothing has been accomplished and yet everything is full to the brim" (to quote Don Juan from Castaneda's books). A line from the poem *Hsin Shin Ming* (Trust in Mind) of the Third Ancestor of Zen also continues to reverberate in my experience: "The more you talk and think about it, the further astray you wander from the truth. Stop talking and thinking, and there is nothing you will not be able to know."

For me, being in the world means that the truth of my existential experience of *dukkha* (unsatisfactoriness or incompleteness), *anicca* (the constantly changing world of phenomena, both internal and external), and *anatta* (lack of an abiding core in any phenomenon, internal or external) become the marker against which all workings of self-deception are tested and found wanting. The ultimate issue in Buddha's teachings is delusion. As we become more and more psychologically sophisticated, we have a greater understanding of the farther reaches of delusion, and, ironically, at the same time open ourselves to its ever-greater complexity. ●

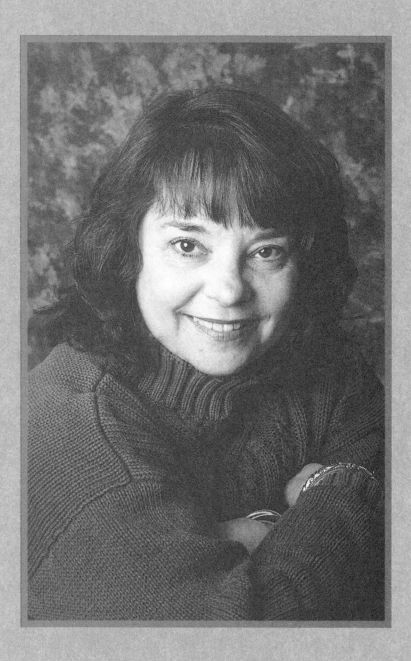

Judith Hanson Lasater

THE SAMADHI OF HERE AND NOW

JUDITH HANSON LASATER, PH.D., physical therapist, and internationally known yoga teacher, has taught yoga since 1971. She is a founder of the Iyengar Yoga Institute in San Francisco as well as *Yoga Journal* magazine. Judith conducts frequent teacher-training sessions in virtually every state and is often a guest at international yoga conventions. • Judith is president of the California Yoga Teachers' Association, as well as the author of numerous articles on yoga and health for national magazines. She is the author of *30 Essential Yoga Poses: For Beginning Students and Their Teachers; Relax and Renew: Restful Yoga for Stressful Times;* and *Living Your Yoga: Finding the Spiritual in Everyday Life.*

ALL I REMEMBER ABOUT MY FIRST YOGA CLASS is
the ceiling. We were in a large room with wooden floors, upstairs at
the Student YMCA/YWCA in Austin, Texas, and the year was 1970.
It was an hour that would change my life, not only by igniting my
love of yoga but also by starting me on the path of a profession I
love: teaching yoga.

At that first class, we were instructed to lie down between each
of the poses and rest. I found that perplexing because we didn't seem
to be "doing anything." Nevertheless, after class I felt refreshed and
more alive, so much so that the next morning I practiced what I
remembered from the class, and have been practicing daily ever since.

What struck me from that first experience, aside from the
conscious resting, was the thought that went through my head
repeatedly during class: "Ah, here is someone (the teacher) who
knows that movement is sacred, that it is a form of worship." Asana,
the yoga postures, felt like a form of worship for me right from the
beginning. This combination of movement and worship was something I had longed for during the Sundays I spent in church
worshipping in more traditional ways. Specifically, I longed for a
deep sense of connection with something beyond myself, some
sense of why I was here on the planet.

In that very first class, specifically during the practice of
savasana, or deep relaxation, I was instructed to watch the flow of
my thoughts. That was a very "new thought" for me, and introduced
to me what I believe is the single most important thing that any
human being can learn. That learning is "I am not my thoughts."

I certainly have thoughts; they tumble forth one after the other endlessly throughout my day, during my practice of asana, and during and as part of my formal seated meditation practice. But lying in *savasana* during that first class, when I was instructed to and in fact started to observe my thoughts, I began to understand on an experiential level that my thoughts and my consciousness are separate. That understanding is the root of the freedom, or *moksha,* that the scriptures teach. That learning was the first of many gifts I have received from my yoga practice.

> **"I have learned that compassion is not something I can do, but is instead something that arises spontaneously in me."**

After I started practicing, I began to search out every book I could find on the topic of yoga. I read practice books written for the general public as well as more esoteric books that were seemingly written in some sort of code for the students of antiquity. After reading many tomes about the various states of *samadhi,* or spiritual wholeness, I made the novice's assumption that I could attain that state of bliss simply by following the "recipe" of asana, *pranayama,* or yoga breathing exercises, and meditation. I hurled myself at the task with enthusiasm and confidence.

I also believed *samadhi* would not be a gradual thing, but instead a sudden and complete transformation. I strove for this state with passion: I held poses for excruciatingly long periods, I chanted, I practiced what I thought was meditation, and I sought out a teacher in India. While I learned a lot "about" yoga, strangely enough, not that much evolved inside me. I became convinced that *samadhi* was not available to me after all. I got caught up instead in raising children and teaching classes, gradually deciding that this lifetime was about different things for me.

Paradoxically, one day while practicing I had an experience of total stillness. "At last! I 'got' it!" I exclaimed. Of course the experience faded in a few minutes, which left me in greater despair. A few weeks later, as I was watching gymnastics class for our children with one of my yoga students, I mentioned this despair. She casually said, "Maybe you are becoming a Buddhist."

Lightning bolts shot through me. Once again I began to study another ancient teaching, to read and practice with fervor. It all felt so familiar. Aside from my intense enthusiasm, what was also familiar was that I still was not immune to getting angry with my husband, impatient with my children, or having thoughts of disappointment in myself. I was caught in the conundrum of believing that I needed to be different, that the way I was right now was not all right. At the same time I was unable to change the way I was, even with devoted spiritual practice.

Eventually I began to understand that it was this very non-acceptance that was keeping me stuck in my patterns. With this awareness about self-judgment continuing to grow in me, slowly I have begun to notice that I have more minutes, and occasionally hours, of ease. I am becoming less quick to judge myself and others. I have learned that compassion is not something I can do, but is instead something that arises spontaneously in me. I have also learned that when I act from the heart of compassion, I help people I will never even meet through the ever-widening circles of compassion that touch person to person.

> "I practice now not so much with
> ambition as with gratitude.
> And I ask myself frequently,
> 'How can I express kindness right
> now?' whether I am in a
> headstand or washing dishes."

Fundamentally I now believe this simple truth to be the bedrock of all religions and spiritual teachings: Choose kindness to self and others.

I still have a daily practice of asana, *pranayama,* and meditation, and probably will for the rest of my life. But I now view these practices not so much as a means to an end but rather as a celebration of my life and spirit. I practice now not so much with ambition as with gratitude. And I ask myself frequently, "How can I express kindness right now?" whether I am in a headstand or washing dishes.

While it might seem strange, what inspires me to practice is my increasing awareness of the fragility and shortness of life. More and more I am acutely aware of the preciousness of this very moment. I am also comforted and reassured when I realize that the strongest force in the universe, like a steel band that can stretch through time and across any distance, is the force of love. Beyond asana and meditation, beyond teaching and parenting and chopping carrots, is the inevitable, invincible, and powerful force we call love. When I remember that, my heart opens and I am alive.

Practice for me now has become the willingness to be present with this grace, this love. I seem to learn this lesson over and over every day: When I do remember to access that awareness, my suffering lessens just a little and my freedom increases by the same amount. Perhaps *samadhi* is given in bite-size pieces after all. ●

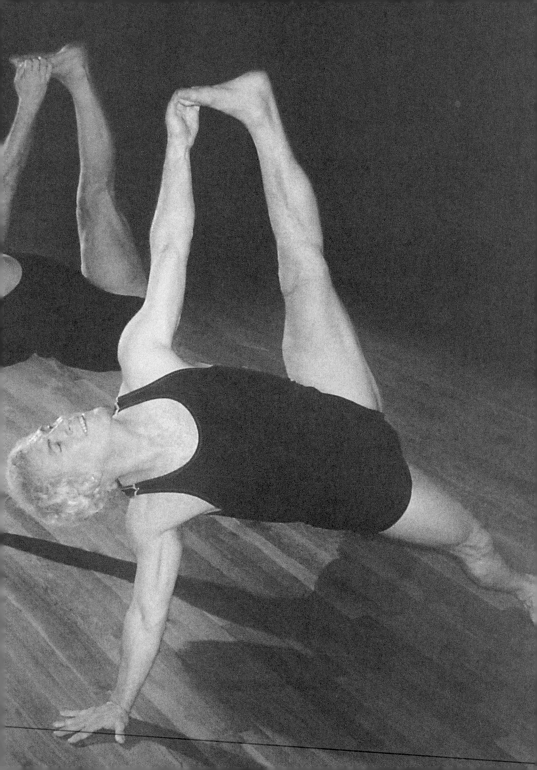

John Friend

ENLIGHTENMENT IN EVERY MOMENT

A seriously playful student of yoga since 1973, **JOHN FRIEND** is one of the most charismatic and respected hatha yoga teachers in the country. With a deep longing to know the mysteries of life, John began a practice of hatha yoga and meditation at age thirteen, including study of quintessential Indian scriptures such as the *Bhagavad-Gita* and the *Upanishads* and later such esoteric subjects as theosophy, wicca, Freemasonry, parapsychology, and quantum physics. • Soon after graduating from Texas A & M University in 1983 with a B.B.A. in finance and accounting, John began his full-time career as a yoga instructor. He studied with a wide range of teachers throughout the '80s, and met his spiritual teacher, Gurumayi Chidvilasananda, in India in 1989. In the early '90s John began teaching seminars throughout the United States and became renowned for his deep knowledge of yoga philosophy and biomechanics, hilarious sense of humor, and open-hearted approach. • In 1997 John founded Anusara Yoga, now one of the fastest growing styles of hatha yoga in the world. Anusara yoga is uniquely transformational in its integration of Universal Principles of Alignment with a life-affirming, heart-oriented Tantric philosophy. John lives in The Woodlands, Texas.

Q. *John, I hope it's all right to start this interview with a personal question. Your mother died recently, and I know that she was an enormous influence and inspiration in both your personal and professional life. From our conversations I know that this and a whole series of other personal losses in the past year must have in some sense drawn you to rely even more deeply upon practice. Loss is an issue that we all must face, and if you're willing, I think it would be helpful to hear your thoughts on the challenges of loss.*

A. Thanks, Stephen, for asking about this, because it has been probably the central theme of my year, and I've been talking about it a lot to my students. I would have to stay this to start with: Through my experience in practice, I've discovered there really is a graceful, supreme spirit that is never absent in my life. Never, never absent. It's really quite amazing, and it's a comfort.

There were many times over the past years when I didn't see it or couldn't feel it, and I doubted that it was really there. I got afraid and became despondent. But what happened so many times was that that spirit would show up, and I'd start to recognize that grace really was there the whole time — carrying me even when I couldn't feel it. So now my response is much more: "Hey, I lost my mother, or I lost a friend, or I lost some money, but I *didn't* lose the core of myself." If I really listened quietly and deeply enough, I experienced that what seemed to be a loss on one side was actually a blessing that was bestowed on the other — the blessing of faith.

Q. *So you really felt held through the whole experience.*

A. I don't want to minimize the pain involved. It definitely was painful, but I didn't lose myself and I didn't lose my vision that life is essentially really good. I sense that there is this great web of pulsating divinity that I'm part of. It's not going to push me away and I'm not going to disconnect from it. So within all the loss, I never really felt absolutely alone. I felt the energy of shakti that constantly infuses me.

When I would share the shakti by speaking to somebody or even just looking at a passerby, I could feel that energy streaming through me, connecting me to the whole world. In those moments I would remember that no matter what is happening, there is a presence that is eternal — a beginningless presence, with me before I was born, with me after this body is dead, a beginningless presence that exists beyond space and time. This whole year has brought me more and more into relationship with that presence.

Q. *The story of your mother's role in your development as a yogi is so interesting and inspiring. Could you talk a little bit about her role in your developing interest in yoga?*

A. Well, she was an intellectual and extremely well-read, so she knew about other cultures and religions and philosophies. When I was very young — even as young as four years old, I think — and certain existential questions would arise, she was able to answer my questions from an unusually broad perspective. As I got a little older she said,

"You know, there's this whole way of being that's practiced, and it's called yoga." She would read me stories of yogis living in the Himalayas that had supernatural powers. As an eight-year-old hearing about guys who could dematerialize and then show up somewhere else — well, they were the greatest superheros you could imagine. It was better than reading a Superman comic book actually!

Q. *It sounds as though she might have been reading to you about Yogananda's experiences.*

A. Yes, and even more esoteric stuff than that if you can believe it! One of the first books she read to me was a collection of short stories. I think it was published by the magazine *Fate.* I don't know if you remember that old magazine: It was called *Fate: Stranger than Fiction.* One of the chapters dealt with the mysterious power of yogis.

She read me a variety of different books like that, dealing with adepts with extrasensory perception and other supernatural powers. From early on I felt that yogis were the ones that knew the answers. That was what sparked me. I started to inquire more into the world of yoga, and of course my mom continued to get me more and more books on Eastern philosophy and yoga. She gave me books by Paramahansa Yogananda, Swami Vishnudevananda, Yogi Ramacharaka, and a lot of others. Of course, *Yoga, Youth, and Reincarnation* by Jess Stearn.

So some of the first books I read were on yoga. By the time I was thirteen, I started going out on my own and getting the scrip-

tures, like the *Bhagavad-Gita* and some of the principal *Upanishads*.
She willingly gave me the money for all of that.

Q. *This is not your run-of-the-mill American mom, is it, John?*

A. No, I guess not! You know that I've developed now a lifelong
interest in the philosophy of Tantra yoga. Well, my mom was the
one who told me about Tantra. More than anything, she lived it. She
said, "Life is good." I'd say, "But, Mom, bad things happen." And
she'd say, "Yes, in this material world you're going to have things we
designate as good and bad, but at the very center of life there is
benevolence. God is good; life is good." She was always looking for
the beauty in things, always looked for the good.

That's been the principal philosophy of my yoga practice.
When you look at a pose when you do this practice, what do you
find? Where do you see the shri in it? Where do you find the beauty
in it? It's already beautiful, inherently. If you want to, then, you can
make the choice to enhance its beauty, take it deeper — but the
beauty is already there.

Q. *I'm sure these powerful life experiences have made an impact on your
practice. How would you characterize your practice these days?*

A. More and more I try to get away from saying, "I do my Puja in
the morning and then I do my asana and some meditation later in
the day." I still do those things, of course, but for me — especially

in the last year — much of my practice is now outside the yoga room. It's yoga off the mat. Rather than "Have I done my asana," my question is now, "How do I interact with everybody?" And then, extending that, how do I relate to nature, how do I look at the trees and the sunset? How do I move and walk? I guess it's fair to say that everything in my day has become my practice.

Of course I still have a regular asana practice. And this attitude also saturates my asana practice. When I do a strong asana practice, I can feel all the effects. Every one of my senses is more refined and enhanced and I'm much more in tune with that pulsating life force. Asana does that for me — it's such a beautiful expression of energy moving through me. Then in meditation I can get so quiet and so deep. Especially lately, when I meditate I feel I'm able to tap into that essence so much more directly than at almost any other time. If I get still and quiet enough, this energy feels as though it's being pooled into me, and in fifteen or twenty minutes I'm saturated with it.

What I want to say is that there is a strong relationship between yoga on the mat and yoga off the mat. I've really come to believe that the energy accumulated in practice has a lot to do with my ability to get clarity about the reality of things. For instance, if my vibratory state is weakened or out of balance, then my ability to gain insight is diminished. When I'm full of energy, full of shakti, and I really set my heart and mind in the right direction with it, then insights come so much more readily.

Q. *Your Tantra training has taught you to place a strong focus in your practice on the relationship between energy and consciousness, isn't that right?*

A. Absolutely right. Tantra is all about the play of energy and consciousness — the dance of energy and consciousness. I'm really, really into this now. In the pursuit of wisdom, it's so easy to leave out the relationship to energy. This can bring a kind of dryness to wisdom, and to a life spent seeking wisdom. Energy brings the juice, the body, the earth — embodiment in every form! Now insight, or wisdom, becomes juicy! Alive. Pulsing with energy and intelligence. Connected to everyday life in the world.

Q. *Whereas some traditions begin directly with an investigation of the mind — citta — my sense, John, is that you're developing an approach that starts with the body — prana, the world of energy.*

A. I love working directly with energy of all sorts. It's such magic. Always such a surprise. I've got to tell you this anecdote: I was just out at a conference in Los Angeles. They had had a big rainstorm and rain had come into this one particular room, a big hall where I was to teach my last class of the day, and soaked the carpet. The teachers that had been teaching in the room all day were complaining, saying, "Look, you can't even breathe in this room, it's horrible." They were all warning me, since I was going to have the biggest class of the day, with the whole room completely filled with about a hundred twenty people.

I came into the room to teach my class and I lit some incense. I had the whole group begin to chant. We started praising spirit, treating this room — complete with its wetness — as a sacred place. Within minutes the air seemed to clear. There was one student who had been taking classes in the room all day who told me later that she had been about ready to vomit by the time I walked in. Well, by the end of the hour class there was so much shakti in the room that you didn't smell any mustiness at all. People were so high that there was a kind of light in the room. This dank, dark-walled place had literally become a temple. It was so tangible that people could see it. They were having incredible heart experiences from the shakti in the room. This is what energy can do if you honor it, appreciate it, recognize it.

Q. *This story sounds like a perfect evocation of the central Tantra view that the whole world is saturated with the divine. In this view, powerful change can be created by just changing where you're standing in relationship to experience.*

A. Exactly. I've really been attempting to be more articulate and poetic in my praise of life and the shakti, trying to invoke her presence more and more. As you say — honoring, recognizing, acknowledging the reality of energy and shakti. I've found that when we live this way, all the different manifestations of creative endeavor that we can choose to do become a kind of collaboration with shakti. Life becomes like one gigantic art project.

For me, we're here to create and to inspire each other. It's uplifting and celebratory. This doesn't mean don't grieve. Yes, grieve! And with this approach you can even get down and grieve fully. It's all part of our total tribute. When I gave the eulogy to my mother in the biggest church in the city, the church was packed. You could hear everyone totally having their heart opened through the celebration of another's life. And, of course, there were so many tears. Those tears were shakti, too.

Q. *So the shakti energy is our source of creativity and transformation?*

A. Yes. And honoring the presence of this divine energy in every being is a way of praying. You can pray when you say "Hey, I like what you're wearing" or "You do a good job at that." You're collaborating in the art project by being the appreciator. Then the shakti gets even brighter and the person is inspired to improve even more. This is why the shakti is important, because it's tangible; it's not just an intellectual thing.

The approach of Vedanta says, "Look, the embodied world isn't real. It is an illusion. The only thing that is real is *brahman,* or consciousness." But Tantra says, "It's real. The world is real. And it's all saturated with the Divine." If you look closely, everything is vibrating with a luster. Divinity has simply taken an endless variety of different colors and forms.

And why? This is the part I love. Divinity is just expressing itself out of its pure love of celebration. In the Tantra philosophy they'd say that the world exists for no other reason than for its own delight. For its own delight!! The universe, consciousness, dances itself into creation just for the sheer fun of it, the play, the self-expression. How wonderful is that?

You do things for no other reason than the delight in doing them. The goal is to have fun, to experience the delight, and to really appreciate that life is dual. You're going to have ups and downs; you're going to have triumphs and losses; you're going to be hurting; there's going to be suffering — and that is not bad, that's just life. By being grounded and recognizing that everything passes, there's a profound joy at the center of things that has always been there — there's no beginning to it and there will be no end to it. It's the energy that moves the supreme dancer. There's no beginning and no end: It's not one big bang that collapses and that's it. It's just one big bang after another.

The goal of practice for me is being able to tap into this joyful way of living — to connect with my heart. In any activity I'm doing, I feel the connection with life and experience the beauty within me. I am in touch with the glory of knowing that there is a supreme consciousness functioning in me even as I do whatever task I'm doing. The whole goal of practice is reveling in and fully participating in and collaborating with that glorious life within me. If one lives in this way, then every moment is a moment of enlightenment. ●

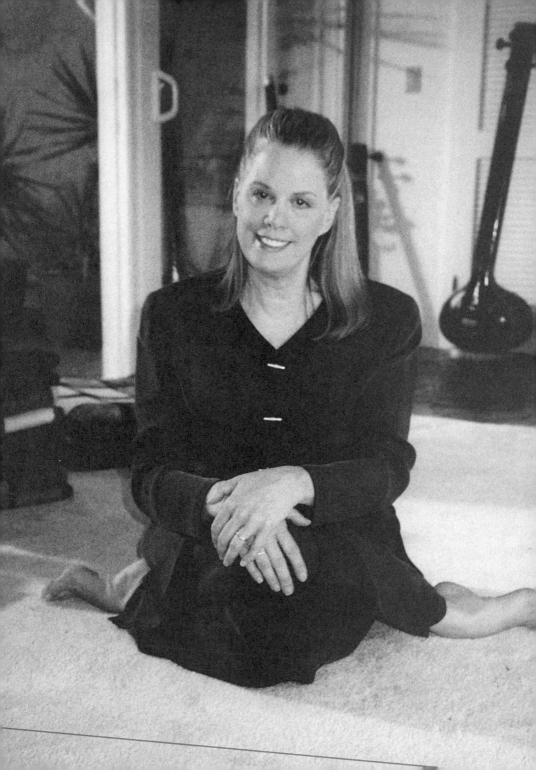

Rama Berch

I ALWAYS BELONGED TO GOD

RAMA BERCH is the founder of Master Yoga Foundation and the originator of Svaroopa® Yoga. In addition, she served as Founding President of the national Yoga Alliance and of San Diego's Yoga Teachers Association. She has been a yoga teacher since 1976. • As a single mother of three, Rama left her successful career as an accountant in California to undertake training in yoga, meditation, healing, massage, and Eastern traditions. After visiting a meditation center in 1976, she received a powerful and spontaneous initiation from a living Master. Traveling to India for a three-week retreat with her Master, Rama recognized that this was what she had always been seeking. She moved into the ashram with her three children to study, practice, and live yoga with her Guru in the United States and India. After eleven years of training, Rama settled in San Diego and has been teaching there since 1987.

I ALWAYS BELONGED TO GOD. And I always loved the world. My problem was that God and the world didn't seem to go together. At church they told me that I had to be "good" to find God, but I loved being bad.

When I was growing up, my favorite books were two big books of Old and New Testament stories with beautiful drawings. I read them over and over. I vividly remember our minister telling a story of Jesus speaking to two brothers in their fishing boat. He looked into their eyes and said, "Come follow me." They did. That minister became my first true teacher when he asked, "What kind of man could have that effect on someone?" I was stunned by my sudden glimpse into who Jesus must have been, and instantly angry that I was living thousands of years too late. I stayed angry at God for years. I wanted someone to look me in the eyes in that way.

I tried to be good. I got married and had children, but I still loved to dance on the wild side. I got divorced and became a bit wilder. I moved from one thing to another quickly, because nothing really worked. I didn't know I was searching, but I was. I tried looking inside myself with psychotherapy. I spent years as a client as well as a student — even got a degree and went on to graduate school. There was no God in it, so I left. I considered becoming a minister but dropped it when I found yoga. I realized then that I wasn't even Christian.

"I have a problem with sin," I said in the meeting I had requested with my minister. "I don't believe myself to be a sinner. I never have." Jack was a new minister, serving as the summer fill-in while our regular minister was on vacation. I added, "Maybe it's a sin to believe that I'm not a sinner. Every Sunday, when I 'confess my sins before God-the-Almighty-Father,' I feel that I am telling a lie. Something deep inside says I'm not a sinner, but the Church keeps telling me I am. I can't continue to come if I have to believe I'm a sinner."

I described the yoga books I'd been reading. "Yoga tells me I am Divine Consciousness. This feels deeply true to me. These books say that I am a perfect manifestation of Divine Consciousness, but that I don't know it, and all I have to do is realize the Truth that already dwells inside. Christianity tells me I'm a sinner and that I need someone else to redeem me before God. I can't stay in the Church if that's what I'm supposed to believe."

Jack had one more year to go in his own training and was willing to start with, "I don't know. Let's look up the word *sin.*" He pulled books off the shelves and checked each index for *sin.* Every book had many entries, but none of them offered a definition. After six or seven books, he opened a really fat dictionary and found the entry. The definition began with, "Sin is separation from God." In delight I shouted, "Yes — *that* I've *got!*"

In that moment I realized that the only thing I had ever wanted was to end that agonizing inner separation. I knew it was yoga that had helped me understand what I'd been feeling all my life. We talked for another hour and he ended by asking me to give the sermon on Sunday. My parents came. I quoted the Bible, the

Upanishads, and the Gurus I'd been studying. I talked about being inspired by the teachings of yoga instead of being downtrodden by feeling that I am a sinner. I invited everyone to think differently of themselves. They all hugged and thanked me as they left. I felt validated and confirmed. It was a new type of confirmation: a confirmation in the faith, but a different faith from before. I never went back to church.

I had an extraordinary dream a few nights after visiting a local meditation center. A wiry dark-skinned Aboriginal man lifted a spear and a long forklike thing. I asked him to wait for a moment. As he waited, I reminded myself, "I am eternal. Even if my body dies, I do not die." Then I was ready. He pierced my heart with the spear. The trident wrapped its two outer tines around my skull as the center one pierced my third eye. Instantly I awoke, startled but not afraid. I shared the story at the meditation center the next week and they told me, "That was Shiva."

"I knew it was yoga that had helped me understand what I'd been feeling all my life."

I chanted to Shiva. I read and studied. Most important, I meditated. Every morning I got up before the sun — and before my three children awoke — and meditated for an hour. As soon as I sat down, the heat of Kundalini climbed my spine and moved me into fantastic yoga poses. I quickly found that if my partner and I had been sexually active the night before, there was no heat, there were no poses — and there was no bliss. I knew what I wanted. Since that time celibacy has taught me more about relationship than anything else ever had. I have never felt that I was giving something up; I was getting so much more on the inside.

> "I love the world and I belong to God.
> I always have, but now I know it."

I went to India and met the Guru who had ignited the fire within me. I looked into his eyes and I knew that this was what I had been searching for. I had waited lifetimes to follow him. I moved in. I became a yoga "nun," or *brahmachari*. I got certified as a yoga teacher, a meditation teacher, a *pranayama* teacher. Then he sent me home. Six weeks later he died.

I fell back into the world, loving and hating it at the same time. I couldn't put it all together — God and the world were still so separate. One day I overheard a conversation between two of my coworkers. It was one of those ordinary conversations, with both of them complaining at length about someone or something. Suddenly, in the droning on, I saw the sutras in full living color. There we were, all living out the teachings of yoga — caught up in the mental chatter while not recognizing our own divinity. It was like waves crashing on the shore for me: I got it.

I went back to the texts and understood them for the first time: This is all God. I went back to India. I started teaching again, but something had changed inside me — the world and God had come together. I love the world and I belong to God. I always have, but now I know it. The practice is called Tantra. I know I still have a long way to go, but the existential angst is gone. The Presence is too present for me to ignore. She's still working on me, but now it's fun! ●

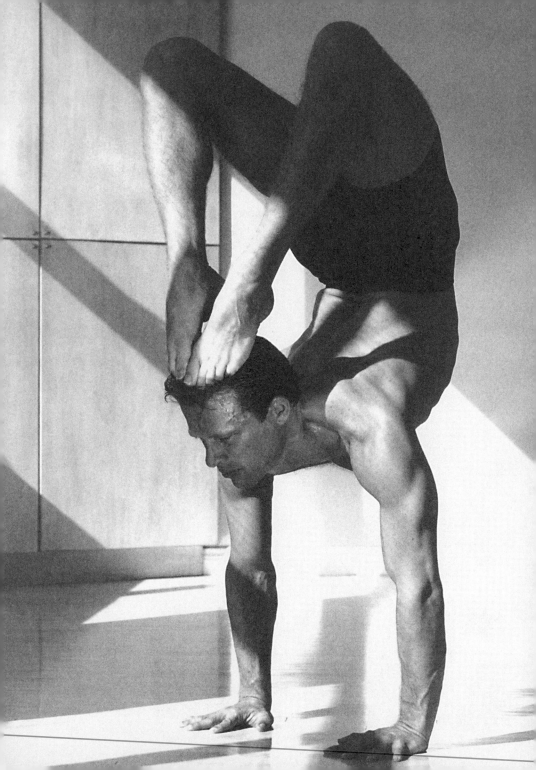

Rod Stryker

A PASSION THAT LED TO THE HEART

ROD STRYKER began his study of yoga at the age of nineteen. Three years later he began an intensive apprenticeship with internationally renowned yoga master Kavi Yogiraj Mani Finger. Rod became a dedicated part of this spiritual lineage that included some of India's leading yoga masters of the past century: Paramahansa Yogananda, Swami Sivananda of Rishikesh, and Ramana Maharshi. Rod became his teacher's only American disciple to be given the title of Yogiraj, master of yoga. • Rod has owned two yoga studios in Los Angeles, Yoga Tantric Institute and Yogatopia. Rod is the creator of Pure Yoga. The mission of Pure Yoga, in Rod's words, is "to inspire and empower individuals to achieve their full physical, emotional, intellectual, and spiritual potential so they may enjoy a richer, more rewarding life. It provides knowledge, wisdom, and tools that enhance all aspects of modern life through the timeless spirit and teachings of yoga." • Rod has developed an array of award-winning video and audio programs including Gaiam's *Peak Performance Yoga* series. He lives in Los Angeles and is father to two sons, Jaden and Theo.

Q. *How did you get started in yoga, Rod?*

A. I, like most people who are drawn to yoga, felt enough discomfort in my life that I longed for it to be more sweet and less painful. It was fate that brought yoga to me. I was twenty years old and had just left college midway through my junior year. I have to thank my mother for that. She was the one who first acknowledged that I was mostly uninspired and uninvolved with school — and she was right.

As a philosophy and psychology major, I found that my only inspiration came from a single professor who taught ancient Greek philosophy. (Aristotle was a revelation.) My mother was the one who said, "If you're not going to take school seriously and apply yourself, you shouldn't go. And if you're not going to go to school, you'll have to pay your own way."

I can tell you that although I wasn't aware of it at the time, her version of "tough love" was one my life's greatest gifts. Abandoning the nest meant confronting myself and, for the first time, my choices. It would be only a few months before they both led me to yoga.

I began working full time at my first legitimate paying job — nothing glamorous: I was a busboy. I resumed doing pottery, a hobby that I loved, and I renewed a relationship with my high school sweetheart. I believe I even had a waterbed at the time. Yes, I was cruising along fairly well, until one warm and windy night when I found her in bed with another man. Very quickly the little

— and I thought wonderful — world I had built around me after I left school seemed to crumble. Racked with the hurt of betrayal and a profound sense of disillusionment, I could not have been more perfectly ripe when, a few weeks later, someone recommended yoga.

Q. *How did you find an instructor back in those days, Rod?*

A. I was in Denver at the time and there was a huge yoga community — one of the largest in the United States — of followers of Guru Maharaji. Quite a few of them worked at the restaurant where I was busing tables. It was there that a waitress said, "Hey, you look tired; you should do yoga." I was too busy to go to her class, so on her recommendation I got *Light on Yoga*.

Reading Mr. Iyengar's introduction — a synthesis of Patanjali's *Yoga-Sutra* and the eight limbs of Ashtanga, essentially the core of yoga philosophy — was an amazing experience. I had the sense that rather than learning something new, I was being reintroduced to an ancient companion, a truth I had known and lived before. The theories were far more accessible than anything I had read in my academic studies. I recall feeling that even reading about yoga reduced the loneliness and despair that had motivated me to reach for it in the first place. Even more exciting, yoga provided something I could do — namely postures — that would help me embody what was inspiring me intellectually. It stoked an ancient fire. I dove into practice.

Q. *You taught yourself postures using* Light on Yoga *as your guide?*

A. I've had a lifelong tendency to throw all of myself into whatever I am passionate about. I was voted most inspirational player on my high school football team — that sort of thing. So, yes, I was self-taught for my first nine months. I was both inspired by some deep calling and, given that I didn't have a teacher, flying by the seat of my pants.

The book, if I remember correctly, offers a seven-year program, describing a specific program for months one through three, then four through six, and the first year, the third year, all the way to a seventh year. The fifth pose listed is *utthita parsvakonasana,* Extended Lateral Angle Pose. Mr. Iyengar recommends a thirty-second to two-minute hold in the posture. Naturally I held it for two minutes. I remember coming out of it on the first side and literally having an epiphany! It's hard even now to find the right words to describe the kind of exhilaration I felt.

Perhaps the most fascinating part of it to me was how bare an experience it was. There I was in my apartment alone, just the wisdom of the pose confronting the confines of my body, mind, and gravity. I was awestruck with the possibilities, the opportunities to expand and challenge myself in the light of something so simple, so complete, and yet so sublime. That all unfolded on the fifth pose.

That first experience moved me enough to practice every day. Almost instantly, and increasingly over the next weeks, I found more energy and vitality and a sense of rest and ease. My difficulties

— the loss of my first love, my psychological baggage, whatever — all seemed to diminish. Every time I practiced I found myself consistently coming back to a place of renewed clarity and freedom.

After a few months into my dedicated practice, I approached the woman who suggested I try yoga to thank her and give her an update on my practice. She was astonished, and mentioned in a very offhand way, "You know, if you can only do two poses, you should do Shoulder Stand and Plow." (I may have mentioned something about the fact that my practice required a lot of time and that it was hard to fit it all in.)

Since Mr. Iyengar said to do Shoulder Stand for between one and thirty minutes, I began doing it for thirty minutes, followed by Plow for fifteen minutes — no preparations, no counter poses. I did this daily, and since practicing was consistently offering more epiphanies, I assumed I was doing something right. Clearly I still had had no formal instruction whatsoever, no direction about what to do, what to look for, nothing. This is the cautionary part of the tale of yoga without a teacher: The way I was practicing was flattening my cervical spine, though it wouldn't affect me until years later.

What kept me coming back to the yoga was that I was having deeply profound experiences in *savasana* — astral experiences, leaving my body, floating over Denver — and mind-boggling experiences of *sunyata* (emptiness) — in spite of not knowing their significance or that they were even something that practitioners aspire to.

Q. *When did you finally begin studying with a teacher?*

A. After almost a year of practicing on my own, I moved back home to Los Angeles. The first person I talked to was one of my best friends from high school, who told me that he had just started doing yoga — kundalini yoga. He invited me to come to class with him. This marked the first time, after practicing for nearly a year, that I worked with a teacher.

I went on to practice kundalini yoga for the next couple of years as a "sporadic fanatic," which meant every day for thirty days and then four times the next month. That's how it went for a couple of years until I decided to get committed. I decided that the next summer I would go to "kundalini yoga camp" for six weeks. It's hard to imagine, but I was giving real thought to "tying the turban": becoming a Sikh. I had actually purchased the material for the headdress — a scary notion now that I think about it.

Just about the time Mom may well have been reconsidering her earlier suggestion that I leave school, providence intervened with its own plan. I met a woman (in a dance club, no less) who would, in a few weeks, take me to a yoga class with Alan Finger. I remember the date was April 10, 1980. I'm not quite sure whatever happened to the would-be turban. In a matter of months I became a disciple of Alan, and of his teacher and father, Kavi Yogiraj Mani Finger.

Mani, who was about seventy-two years old when I met him, was an extraordinary and powerful being. He was South African, definitely Western, yet a direct disciple of some of India's greatest teachers of the past century: Paramahansa Yogananda, Swami Sivananda of Rishikesh, and the great mystic, Tantric master, and linguist Bharati, who was known as the "Shakespeare of India" because he had translated all of Shakespeare's writings into Hindi.

I still think of Mani as my spiritual father. Alan provided practical wisdom and experience of his father's teachings, as well as additional guidance. Together they initiated me into the ancient tradition of Tantra, the probable source of yoga, and arguably its most comprehensive and sublime approach. Tantra yoga integrates physical postures, breathing, yogic meditation and energy cultivation techniques, Ayurveda, and a seemingly endless body of diverse practices born from a distinctly nondualistic worldview. Its ultimate intent is to empower practitioners to thrive in all areas of life. The word *tantra* means "to weave." Its central theme is the weaving of spiritual experience and everyday life into a single, vibrant tapestry.

Tantra is distinct from classical yoga, in part because it is nondual. It aspires to and provides the means by which we merge spirit (non-matter) and the world (matter). It sees the infinite not separate from, but within, the finite. This life-affirming philosophy was counter to everything that I had assumed and studied up to that point. It was both a revelation and a relief from my philosopher's mind.

My teachers stressed that yoga without meditation isn't yoga. Within a few weeks I had started a daily meditation practice, doing a specific personal practice under my teachers' guidance. As I meditated, I found myself learning and stretching in ways that the movement of my body or the machinations of my mind had never revealed. For the first time, really, I found a home in my heart.

As I look back, meditating daily for twenty-five years, coupled with the blessing of such extraordinary mentors in my life, more than anything else has helped develop whatever is positive about me as a man, teacher, father, citizen, or whatever. Soon after I began to meditate, I became hungry to teach. On June 23, 1980, I taught my first yoga class.

Q. *You know, one of the ten qualities of enlightened mind in Buddhism is strong determination, or "resolve" — the willingness to dive into the dharma, or path, with both feet. It sounds as though that's a quality you've always had, Rod.*

A. That may be true. But it was not until I was blessed and guided by a master into the path of meditation that I felt passion quickening my dharma. Prior to that I knew strong determination, but it didn't necessarily bring me any closer to inner or outer peace.

Q. *Looking back now, over the years, how would you say that yoga has transformed your life?*

A. With the benefit of time, I can look back and recognize how much fear played a central role in my life. Even though, from what I hear anyway, I appeared really "cool" in high school, inside it was a very different story. In real terms, before yoga I was much more inhibited, shy, and withdrawn. My choices were informed less by trust, faith, and inner strength. Yoga and meditation helped bring out more of the best of Rod.

Over time, my commitment to the contemplative practices of yoga helped uproot the subtle plague of fear. Practice also fortified and expanded my joy, my celebration of life. That may be somewhat counterintuitive, because conventional wisdom says that yoga quiets you down and as a result neutralizes personality. For me it did the opposite. It has empowered me, made me more courageous and enthusiastic about life.

Perhaps most meaningful to me has been the effect it has had on my relationship to spirit. I grew up without any formal religious or spiritual training. Incredibly, without any direct influence from my teachers, practice slowly revealed a deeper truth. What evolved naturally, in its own time and way, was an ever-stronger sense of the Divine. Years of meditation increasingly have illuminated a visceral sense of a creator — a permanent, loving, and benign Source. What evolved for me is the awareness of that Source reminding me of the sweetness, profundity, and possibility of life.

What drew me to be a psychology and philosophy major was an indwelling hunger to know. I have always sought to understand the depth and possibility of human potential. What are we, as human beings, here to do? What are we capable of? From saints and philosophers to artists, what, in the highest sense, determines a life well lived? A part of me knew that if I were to live fully, powerfully, authentically, having the right answers to these questions was essential. I just didn't know how or where to find them.

Until I found meditation, I did not know *prajna* (the inner voice), the wisdom of the heart. Without it, from a very young age, I turned to my intellect and became cerebral, assuming that thinking could provide all the answers. Meditation and the grace of a spiritual lineage helped me discover a knowing that I had been trying in vain to uncover through thinking. Prior to having that knowing, a real sense of freedom eluded me.

The treasure of being emboldened began to percolate in those very first yoga experiences, but it's only after years of practice that it has reshaped me. Now I can't imagine life without the gifts that practice has afforded me.

Q. *Can you talk a little bit about who, in particular, has inspired you in your practice?*

A. Throughout my life my "beacons" have been anyone that I felt was able to combine both a spiritual and a fervent embrace of life. In early childhood, my biggest hero was Leonardo da Vinci. Growing up we had a book of his — a canon of all his science, art, drawing, and engineering — that I would pull off the shelf. Turning page after page, I would just stare, probably hoping that through osmosis I could learn to be limitlessly adventurous and creative.

That is one of the things that first attracted me to my teacher of the past four years, Pundit Rajmani Tigunait, Ph.D. "Punditji" is the spiritual head of the Himalayan Institute and successor to Swami

Rama of the Himalayas. He utterly embodies the highest in sublime ideals coupled with ease, humor, and an enterprise and practicality in his approach to daily life. He's a husband, father to two children, and at the age of fifty-four holds two Ph.D.s and has authored twelve books. His creative vibrancy is contagious. He's certainly a tremendous source of inspiration to me.

So is *sri vidya* — Tantra's most comprehensive approach to practice — the tradition in which Punditji is a master and into which he has initiated me as a teacher. Within days of beginning my work in this tradition, I realized that my first twenty years of practice and study were preparation for our relationship and my work in *sri vidya*.

Both my teachers, Mani (who passed on in the summer of 2000) and Punditji, raised their voices if needed, and yet both have such gentleness. Mani smoked Cuban cigars and would enthusiastically quote William Blake at the dinner table. He translated the Vedas, lived in India at Sivananda's ashram in Rishikesh, and unabashedly wore expensive jewelry. He loved his family. He loved to talk politics. Punditji's style is different, but both have taught me as much over dinner as when they were teaching me esoteric Tantric science. Both have been spectacles of exuberance and lightheartedness, intensity and commitment, unwavering strength and courage. I've never seen either afraid, yet both have not hesitated to reveal their humanity.

Tantra captivated me because I longed to understand — even master — the discipline that could produce and encourage this kind of roaring, dynamic personality. Deep down I think that's all I really wanted to be, and I still aspire to be. Teachers leave legacies. My teachers' legacies have been an appreciation of living life to the fullest and an unwavering desire to shine in that living.

Q. *So it's the intensity of Tantra that you admire and are inspired by?*

A. In part, but it's more than just its intensity that is inspiring. Tantra is the one spiritual tradition I have found that celebrates the creator as much as creation, and creativity as a part of — not separate from — spirit. This worldview — that the world is an embodiment of beauty and joy — transformed me. It still does. It's a constant revelation, empowering and inspiring me.

Rabindranath Tagore, the painter, dancer, musician, poet, playwright, and Nobel laureate, was a shining example of Tantra. His accomplishments speak volumes. So does Swami Rama's description of Tagore in *At the Eleventh Hour,* Punditji's biography of Swami Rama. Swami Rama spent time with Tagore at Tagore's ashram and said of him: "Tagore was surrounded by a vibrant tranquility rather than the inner peace that characterizes so many swamis . . . One thing that bothered Swami Rama about some holy men was that it seemed they spent a great deal of their mental energy protecting their heavy load of peace."

The gift of studying with Punditji and Mani is that both shone with that vital spirituality, enlivened by a powerfully creative and elegant love of life. The dynamism of their presence, coupled with the blessings I've received through practice, is the compelling force of my life.

Q. *What has been the role of physical practice postures these days, Rod?*

A. From the mid-eighties to the mid-nineties, I become a very earnest student of asana. But while I learned from and was inspired by many great hatha yoga teachers, in the end I learned that asana is a way of alleviating the symptoms of stress, not its root causes.

My experience was that I would do asana and it would definitely open the door to increased freedom. In my twenties I had plenty of time to practice: two to two and a half hours, seven days a week. So the door would swing open, and yet within twenty-four hours the door would subtly close again. I'd go back to the mat and the door would swing open, only to close again. The real solution to the swinging door had to take place below the surface of my body.

I know now more than ever that if we are to realize yoga's potential, asana must be skillfully combined with meditation, spiritual practice, self-study, and a transformative worldview. This vital synthesis is what inspired me to develop Pure Yoga. In Pure Yoga, posture, breath, and intention are alchemy for the primary purpose of awakening *tejas* (inner light), or "the radiant splendor of personality that expresses itself in love, compassion, creative action, and a melting tenderness that draws all hearts."

Q. *What is the cutting edge of your practice now?*

A. All of the above. There are three edges of my practice, addressing mind, life, and soul. Mental practices include deep reflective practices from the vedic tradition that come under the heading of *jnana* yoga (yoga of knowledge) and are intended to dissolve the subtle fragments of our patterning and unconscious impressions.

At the level of soul, I play at that edge where the world of matter, *nama* (name), and *rupa* (form) dissolves into the realm of supreme bliss and power. However, I am judicious about how far I go into that realm because my main focus is being in the world and embodying to students, to friends, and in particular to my two sons the twin aspects of soul: *avatar* (wisdom) and *prem* (love).

As far as life is concerned, I am only interested in fulfilling the uniqueness of my life by contributing as much as I can to others with the time I have here on this earth.

Among the teachings of Tantra that I am constantly informed by are its references to nature — evocative references that shed light on the awakened state. Nature, it points out, is constant aspiration. Trees grow toward the light, salmon swim upstream, hummingbirds flap their wings ninety times a minute. Earth is not an inert place. It's endlessly dynamic, full of life and liveliness.

I believe that dharma is getting closer and closer to embodying our unique aliveness. The brilliance of practice is that it helps me disentangle myself from all the things that would inhibit me from being my unique aliveness fully. This is what practice has come to mean to me: a way of knowing the beauty of the sublime and the process of rendering me more capable of expressing that beauty as exquisitely as possible in the world. ●

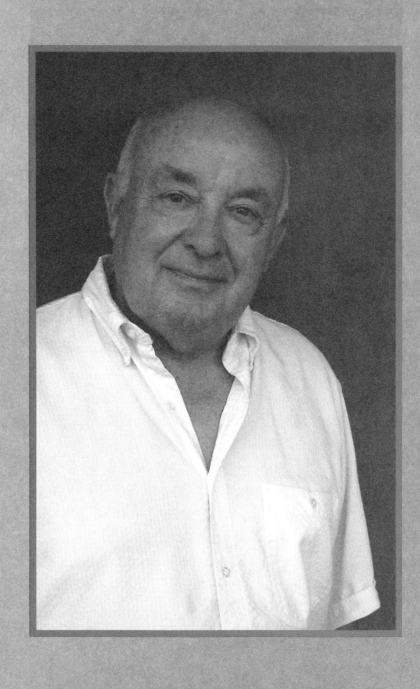

Robert Hall

TRUSTING THE INNER VOICE

ROBERT HALL, M.D., is a psychiatrist and physician of the body/mind, a lay Buddhist priest, a performer, a poet, and a meditation teacher. Once a student of Fritz Perls and Ida Rolf, Robert has been an innovative pioneer in the integration of bodywork, psychotherapy, and Vipassana meditation. • In 1970 Robert cofounded the Lomi School and Counseling Clinic, a clinical training institute for psychotherapists in Santa Rosa, California. Robert was ordained as a lay Buddhist priest and has taught meditation since 1980. He is currently on the teaching council at Spirit Rock Meditation Center in Woodacre, California. He has a published book of poems, entitled *Out of Nowhere.* He has produced two spoken-word CDs: *Out of Nowhere,* with percussionist Brian Hand, and *What a Mystery,* with master composer Teja Bell. Most recently, *Downpour Resurfacing,* a documentary film on his healing methods, was produced by Frances Nkara and screened at the Sundance Winter Film Festival 2003. In the same year, the Ann Arbor Film Festival presented *Downpour Resurfacing* with Most Promising Filmmaker and Lawther/Graff No Violence awards. • Robert is founder of El Dharma Retreats and makes his home in Todos Santos, BCS, Mexico.

Q. *Robert, how has your meditation practice changed your life?*

A. I can't imagine life without spiritual practice. It's been the center of my life for many years. My formal practice started in 1969 with my apprenticeship with Fritz Perls. I also started bodywork and yoga that same year. The very first time I sat down to meditate in a big easy chair in my bedroom, I remember feeling relieved to know what I needed to do at last. It was like coming home. Practice has been that way for me ever since. It inspires my life and it's where I go for answers and direction. It's been the center of my relationships. It gave me the sense of possibility that life could be lived without so much anxiety. At the time I began practice, I was an anxious person and practice was an antidote. The anxiety didn't go away, but I could see how practice diminished it right from the beginning.

Q. *Who inspired you on the path of practice?*

A. I had a number of teachers in my early days, a very rapid succession of incredibly powerful teachers who picked me out. I wasn't even seeking them. It seemed that they found me. They were very magical meetings.

At the age of fifteen my practice began in an unorthodox fashion. No one in my family went past the eighth grade and we were very poor. My father — who was then a janitor in the nearby hospital — managed to get me into the good graces of our family doctor, who was also a surgeon. So when other kids were out playing, I was on the surgical unit learning to assist in surgery. He taught me to take out an appendix and how to assist in a gallbladder operation. I was so small that I had to stand on a box next to the operating room table. Fascinated with the human body, I had rare and wonderful opportunities to see what it looked like inside. It's beautiful: purple, blue, silver, shimmering, and always in motion.

By the time I got into medical school, I had studied every nook and cranny of the body. It took me a long time to discover I wasn't interested in the body itself, but rather in what enlivens it. After training as a psychiatrist, I somehow wound up as a major in the Army, training first-year residents in psychiatry. That's when I met Fritz Perls. Or he met me.

Q. *How did you first encounter Fritz Perls?*

A. It was 1967. He was a maverick psychoanalyst and wild man who was doing dream work at Esalen Institute in California. The night I was there, a very shy woman got up to work on a dream in which she was Eliza Doolittle from *My Fair Lady*. In minutes she went from being painfully shy to belting out "The rain in Spain stays mainly in the plain." Sitting in the audience, I was astonished. Immediately I thought to myself: "I want to know what he knows."

A couple of weeks later, Perls got up and walked over to me in the Esalen dining room. I stood and looked into his eyes and the next thing I knew we were embracing one another and he was saying, "I want you to come and work with me." That's how it happened. I wasn't looking for a teacher and yet he showed up. My whole life has been like that; everything appears. It's just magical.

Perls taught us to be present: That life happens at no other time than here and now. In order to be fully present we have to be free of any unfinished physical, mental, or emotional business. So the work was clearing anything that was an obstacle to being present.

Landing on the hot seat in Perls' group one day, I remember looking into his eyes and beginning some aimless chatter. The next thing I knew my hands were bleeding and there was broken furniture everywhere. I had gone into a rage because of what was locked inside me. That release was the beginning of my path. I was ecstatic.

Q. *You also studied with Ida Rolf, I believe?*

A. Yes. At the same time that I was working with Fritz, I was also apprenticed to Ida Rolf, the mother or founder of Rolfing and Structural Integration. I was the first person she ever trained to do her work, because I was a doctor and she wanted to be legitimate. I was terrified of her. Although she was a very tough lady, she also had a big heart.

Working on me deeply, she altered something; it wasn't just my body, it was my being that got altered. In one session, as she sank her knuckles deeply into the inside of my leg, something happened that revealed in a gut-wrenching way how the body is the pathway to truth. All of a sudden I started seeing ropes. Then scenes flashed by. I was locked in a dark room. I was nude and very young and somebody was doing painful things to me. I felt totally humiliated, but I didn't know what was happening. These visions were incredibly vivid and unquestionably real.

Later, when whoever it was left me there, I tried to put my clothes on, but I didn't yet know how to dress myself. I had both legs in one of the pants holes of my underwear and I kept falling down. I collapsed in humiliation, weeping because of my helplessness. Just at that moment (and this is my first real spiritual experience), a shaft of light came through the window, and I heard my name being called. I looked up and there was a face in the window. I knew that I had been saved.

After that session I went home and called my mother to verify events. She said to me, "Why do you want to remember?" When I was three or four years of age, my brother was born, and I'd run away from home because I didn't want anybody new in the family. As it turned out, after I ran away I had been abducted off the street. Just like that. I had been kidnapped and missing for several days. There had been an overnight search party looking for me, and the face in the window was my father's best friend, who discovered me in that shack.

Growing up I had no idea this had happened. Psychologically unsophisticated, my family thought it best to forget about it. My mother said that I didn't speak for a year afterward. Finally understanding this helped me piece together facts about my life in later years that I could never understand. For example, why I was often terribly frightened, even though I was a psychiatrist and doing very well in life.

Q. *Who introduced you to the Eastern traditions?*

A. There came a point when I became really depressed. I had left Fritz Perls and Ida Rolf and yet this stuff was still teeming inside me. One day at a friend's house I picked up a mimeographed piece of paper with the teachings of a spiritual teacher in India. The teachings spoke very clearly to me. I took the information home and showed it to my then wife, who said, "Well, that's it, isn't it." We called the phone number at the bottom of the sheet and lo and behold, it was our next-door neighbor. We had just moved into this house and I was thinking I would really like to meet this neighbor who had a geodesic dome, and it turned out that when we dialed the number on the sheet, that's who answered. He had just come back from being with a spiritual master in India.

Q. *Who was the spiritual master?*

A. Charan Singh. Picture a mixture of Santa Claus and Genghis Khan dressed in a white gown, with a white turban and a long white beard. We met him in India in 1968. After several months I was initiated into a practice called Surat Shabd yoga, the yoga of sound current. The key practice was meditation, attuning to inner sound, or *shabd,* the sound of the life force. The Sufis call it "The Guest," the "Holy Spirit," or the "wee small voice of God."

While in India I also came under the tutelage of Charan Singh's physician, Randolph Stone, who is the father of polarity therapy. He started teaching me to work energetically with touch and movement, in a healing energy kind of way. I became an apprentice of his for several years both in India and here in the United States. He told me I was his son and he would always be with me, and he always has been. He was eighty-something at the time.

Q. *How did your meditation practice affect your professional direction?*

A. I had been with Fritz Perls for a couple of years as his apprentice and he was grooming me for teaching in Europe. I realized that I wasn't ready to do that. I was a Gestalt therapist, starting out a practice in Structural Integration — integrating mind and body in my work. I hadn't yet really realized the unity of mind/body, though the potential for it was all there in the work I was doing: I did the Gestalt classes at night and bodywork during the day. It was really the meditation practice that brought it all together in a very cohesive way. It healed a split inside.

I've been practicing sound meditation now for thirty-five years. I recently discovered that many advanced Theravadan monks do this same practice, only they refer to it as *nada* practice — listening to the inner sound of silence. The sound comes in very clearly when the mind is peaceful. Surrendering to the sound is basically surrendering to yourself. Much later, what became clear in my Vipassana practice was that the sensations of the body are manifestations of sound in the material world. The sensations are sound. It's just that that's how they show up in this level of consciousness.

Q. *Are you still involved with Singh as your teacher?*

A. That's a long story. Soon it became clear that in order to open my heart and continue on my path, I needed to live with a man — to be intimate with a man. It was a very difficult period for me, but there wasn't any question about it. There was something about that business in my past that was terribly unfinished. I needed intimacy with men, and I knew it.

While teaching bodywork to psychotherapists at the University of Hamburg, I got a chance to see my spiritual master. There was a huge assembly in Wiesbaden and I went to hear him talk. At one point a young Dutch woman came up to the microphone and said, "Maharaji, some of us are wondering about homosexuality." Angrily he interrupted her and said, "I condemn it, do your meditation." Then she said, "But Maharaji, some of us — " And he repeated, "I condemn it, do your meditation." The silence was stunning; never had he made a statement like that before.

I went back to my hotel room and wept. After ten years of relationship, I thought, "What am I going to do?" In the middle of this grief I started hearing the words "You're condemned, you're condemned." Then I thought, "Big deal; so I'm condemned." I started singing "I'm condemned" and I danced around the hotel room. Returning to Hamburg the next day, I noticed the birds were singing and the sun was shining. And our relationship was over.

When you're in love with a guru you have to get up and leave at some point or you don't grow. It's the same as when you grow up and leave your parents' home. Besides, Singh had always said he wasn't the master; sound was. Still I continued the practice.

Q. *How, then, did you get involved in Vipassana, a Buddhist meditation technique?*

A. In 1974 I lived in Mill Valley, California, with my children, and in my home I had a practice of psychotherapy and bodywork. I became known as a person who knew how to fix bad backs. Joseph Goldstein was just returning from India and in the course of his culture shock his back had gone out. His friends brought Joseph to me to work on his back. There was an immediate rapport and friendship that exists to this day. Through the relationship with him I went to Naropa Institute that first summer in 1974 when Chogyam Trungpa, Rinpoche, and Ram Dass were there.

Q. *Robert, especially given the many fantastic and seemingly "fated" meetings with masters throughout your life, you must have thought about the question of karma. How do you explain your remarkable life's course?*

A. The whole thing is a mystery. It all just appeared. I have always felt guided. I have been a fearful sort of person, but in the midst of all there's always been this guidance and a sense of certainty when decisions had to be made.

Q. *How do you tune into this guidance?*

A. In meditation. Through the sound current. I talk to whoever is in there. I think I became aware of my inner voice because there was so much abuse in my childhood. There was so much pain that it tuned me into the inner life early on. Long before I came in contact with Buddhism, my approach was focusing internally — in fact, I thought I had invented it. Then I realized the Buddha beat me to it.

Q. *What is the primary focus of your practice now?*

A. Making my practice constant, allowing practice to fill every day. When I'm not teaching retreats I seem to be practicing constantly. I'm sixty-nine and I have come to realize what's really important in life. For me it's continuous practice, whether I'm in conversation with someone or walking down the street. I take a lot of walks and I practice walking meditation. It's meditation in action in a very real sense, infused with *metta,* or lovingkindness.

My path revolves around the body, learning to find happiness in my skin. The question of how to live and flourish in this physical form is one of my chief concerns. When I learned Vipassana meditation years ago, I was overjoyed, because I understood that I could continue to pay attention to sensations just as I had before.

I hear *shabd,* the inner sound all the time. No matter what I'm doing, it's in the background so I can tune into it at any given moment for guidance or grounding. It has become synonymous with body sensations — that inner *shabd.* So there is a kind of here-and-now touchstone that my body has become. Meditation in action is really body awareness, an inner sound practice that is constant and never goes away. My attention wanders but as soon as I remember, it's immediately present. In Sufi lore it's also referred to as "The Comforter."

When I'm sitting in an airport waiting for a transatlantic flight that I'd rather not take, I really lean on that comforter. Or when I'm alone in the middle of the night and can't sleep, that's where I rest. Guidance comes through the sound current. I talk to whoever is in there, and I feel divinely taken care of.

Q. *Do you still practice psychotherapy?*

A. I do a little bit of therapy in my private practice in Todos Santos in Mexico. I have several clients, but mostly I've lost interest in psychotherapy. It isn't compelling to me anymore. After you've witnessed the human drama, it's just one story repeated over and over again. I'm tired of watching people who make themselves suffer and choose not to listen to any reasoning about it. I can see that we're all compelled to do what we do. What I am interested in is being directly involved in each moment and witnessing how it unfolds.

Q. *How can we lessen our suffering?*

A. If we can flow from moment to moment, then life is good. But when we fix on a certain detail and can't let go, that's where suffering comes in. Most recently I was sitting in a retreat where Sylvia

Boorstein was teaching. Having sat for thirty days, I was due to teach the next month. Soon I started comparing myself to others: "I don't know anything. All my colleagues are so good, and I've been faking it all this time. It's over; what am I going to do?" The Buddha calls this practice "me-making."

It sounds funny, but the suffering was horrible. I couldn't sleep, couldn't eat, had no peace — thinking, thinking — until finally I thought: *metta, metta, metta*. I started working with those beautiful *metta* phrases: "May I be free from suffering, because there has been enough suffering." I worked it for a long time and then all of a sudden there was a voice in my head that said: "Yes, you may be free of suffering." And the suffering was gone.

One of those ordinary times followed, except that the awareness of love now filled me inside and out. Remembering that the Buddha taught only two things, suffering and the end of suffering, I truly felt blessed, because I had the experience of knowing that there is an end to suffering.

Experiences come during practice if you sincerely want to let go and discover what's true. Sometimes they're ecstatic, the kind Sylvia Boorstein calls "bells and whistles." And sometimes they're ordinary. But afterward I realize that what makes any of them special is that there isn't any "me" there. There is a ceasing of the point of view of "self": that I am a separate person, or that you are other than me. I have come to realize that I don't know what enlightenment is, but if it's anything like a full-time experience of that, I'm definitely signing up. ●

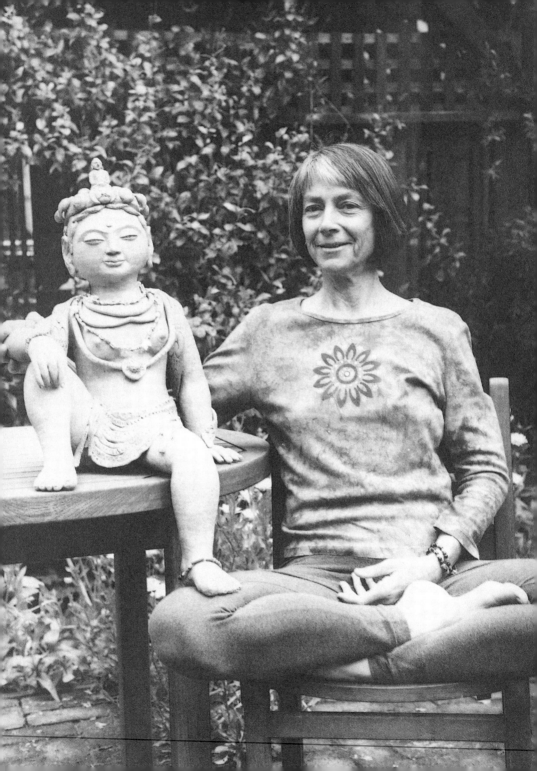

Patricia Sullivan

DHARMA GATES ARE BOUNDLESS

PATRICIA SULLIVAN began her yoga practice in 1970, studied in India with B. K. S. and Geeta Iyengar in the '80s, and taught teachers in training at the San Francisco Iyengar Yoga Institute through the late '90s. She has taught nationally and internationally for over twenty-five years. Yoga has guided her life decisions since the beginning of her practice, as she became aware very early on that the life of a nine-to-fiver was not for her. Working part time for many years just to make ends meet, Patricia spent the majority of her time honing her practice and teaching of yoga and her imagination and craft as a sculptor. • Patricia's curiosity about yoga and the mystery of life has led her to explore a variety of pathways and moved her deeper into her practice. In her teaching, she guides students toward greater and greater sensitivity to the results of their actions on body, mind, and spirit, both in the context of yogic practices and in daily life and relationships. • Patricia lives in Northern California with Edward Espe Brown. They colead Zen and yoga retreats nationally and internationally.

Q. *How did you get started with yoga, Patricia?*

A. I took an initiation at the age of twenty in Surat Shabd Yoga. Part of the deal was that I had to promise to meditate two hours a day. I was given a mantra and told all these inspiring stories about blissful experiences. Of course, nothing really happened for me. I did give it an honest try for a little while but, actually, I just couldn't meditate for two hours a day.

Q. *What is Surat Shabd Yoga?*

A. It's one of the sound schools of yoga. By internally chanting the mantra you were given you were to open yourself up to hearing the internal sound. You were encouraged to be vegan — they didn't have that word, as I recall, but you were not to eat meat, fish, or eggs, or anything that contained any of those things. The people that were really, really thin were the ones that were held in greater esteem.

Q. *And what was it that brought you to that level of deep practice at the tender age of twenty?*

A. A handsome young man. What else?! He had given me *An Autobiography of a Yogi* and, of course, that book is filled with mystical experiences, so this encouraged me. Within a few months of initiation, someone else gave me the book *Yoga, Youth & Reincarnation,* and there were wonderful mystical stories in that book as well. There were some drawings of yoga postures, too, so I started doing Sun Salutation and yoga postures. That was the beginning of my relationship with yoga.

Q. *How did this exposure to yoga change your life at the time?*

A. It was the 1970s. I had smoked some marijuana. I had taken a number of acid trips. Like so many of us, I had experienced something *other* than what I was raised to do, which was to go to college and find some good, stable career. Somehow I knew that I didn't want to do any of those more mainstream kinds of things. So when I experienced yoga, I thought, "Hmm, this is something that might take me down a road that will be different from all that."

I had already had what you might call "the empty successful accomplishment experience": I was able to get straight A's in school; I got on the cheerleading team; I did some of those things that get you into "the in crowd." And I discovered early on that it just wasn't satisfying. I guess you could say that from a young age, I was already dissatisfied — and fortunately I didn't think I had to try harder at that same old approach to life. I *am* the kind of person who thinks I have to try harder, but at least I didn't think that I ought to go down that same path again and again. It seemed to me that something needed to be different.

Yoga pointed me in a different direction very quickly. When I started doing asana, the yoga postures, I had a very strong feeling of many unnecessary things dropping away — especially tension and inadequacy. Having smoked marijuana and taken acid trips and rebelled in so many other ways, I had already let go of "I'm going to look like the rest of society in my life." I was ripe for yoga.

Q. *Did you continue to go deeper in your study of yoga?*

A. I enjoyed a kind of freestyle life for a couple of years in Hawaii and then a crisis erupted — I had to have an appendectomy. Well, it was actually a misdiagnosis, and though I did have the procedure, it turned out that I didn't really need to have had it. But it was good karma anyway. As it turned out, I didn't have enough money to pay for the operation. After I had come out of the anesthesia and could talk, there appeared this social worker at my bedside, saying basically, "OK, now we're going to have to apply for welfare to pay for this."

My first response was that I certainly wasn't going to call my parents for help. But then I thought, "OK, I do need something. I need to find some other way to live. This lifestyle won't do for the long haul." The appendectomy crisis woke me up to that. Prior to that incident, my parents had been repeatedly saying to me, "If you want to go back to college, we'll support you. Look for something you might like to do." So I did.

I went back to college. But I'd fortunately already been initiated into asana, into yoga, so I kept that with me as I went through my college experience, and it became an essential companion. I did two years in dental hygiene and got a certification that allowed me to become licensed as a dental hygienist. The reason I chose that was because it was only a two-year program, and my very practical Capricorn side said, "In two years you will be able to have a job — a high-paying job at which you will need to work only two or three days a week."

After dental hygiene school, I picked up a pencil one day on the beach and started drawing. Suddenly another interest came in, and fortunately I made room for it. I discovered this passionate artistic side that I wanted to explore as well.

I practiced dental hygiene part time, but it allowed me to pursue practicing yoga and my artwork without having to worry about earning a living from those two passions. I didn't have to get them involved in the money side of life.

Q. *How did your yoga practice help in your work as a dental hygienist?*

A. It's interesting how that worked out. I don't know if you're familiar with Swami Chetanananda. He's a teacher of Kashmiri Shaivism, which is also referred to as kundalini yoga. He teaches, as many teachers do: "Don't try to escape the world. You need to be part of the world and to bring your practice into it." I've had that orientation with both my yoga practice and my art all along. It turns out I was really able to bring my practice into my work in the most surprising way.

It was very interesting how the two fit together. I found that as a result of my practice I could offer a kind of presence to the dental patients in our office so that often they didn't need to have anesthetic when they worked with me. I could help them be with fear, or pain, or discomfort. I was able to be a quiet, calm, gentle presence right at their sides — and that takes away a lot of pain. This gave me a confidence that I didn't have initially that people actually can calm themselves and come into a very different state of mind. My experience with patients actually gave me the courage to teach.

I enjoyed the people connection of the work, but the physical tedium and the repetition were not great. Luckily I had the flexibility to have to work at it only two days a week, but even those two days were difficult and draining. I think my yoga practice saved me from insanity during those years. When I came home from work, drained from supporting others, I would be made whole again through practice.

I didn't eat dinner until 7:30 or 8:00 in the evening so I could have a long session of asana practice. That hour and a half that I would have before dinner saved me. I used to say to my roommate, "I think I'd be an alcoholic if it weren't for this, for something to whip this tension away." Most jobs that you do for eight hours a day, even if it's just a sedentary job, can take their toll.

Q. *What does your practice look like these days?*

A. Well, it's definitely modified a lot through the years. These days I'm beginning with a couple of asanas. I often start by just sitting on my heels — I don't sit in *vajrasana* with my heels apart — and use a blanket to relax my calf and hamstring muscles. Then I'll do an *upavista konasana,* the Seated Wide Angle Pose. And then, actually, I just sit in meditation. Sometimes I come in and straightaway sit in meditation. I'll sit for half an hour or forty-five minutes and that often includes some *pranayama.*

More and more I find that I just look for what I'm needing on that particular day, in that particular moment. I'm not forcing anything. Often I'll do an awareness kind of breathing, *nadi shodhana* — switching my awareness from left to right. It's amazing how just taking the awareness away from the side that's more available to the side that's kind of shut down actually shifts the attention into a deeper space, because, of course, you have to pay a lot more careful attention to feel what's not easily accessible. Then it's so natural to let myself slip into some quiet time. If my mind is stirred, I might use a mantra, something simple like *"so ham."* Or sometimes in those quiet times I invoke Ganesha.

Q. *It sounds as though much of the focus of your practice these days is really on stillness.*

A. The focus is on staying grounded and connected. This experience of being grounded is very important to me. I've always needed a connection to practice to be able to maintain this grounded feeling, and to be in the world. I'm fairly relaxed in my teaching now, but basically I'm rather shy. I'm not necessarily hermit-like, but I'm happy to spend a lot of time alone. I like to do my sculpture, which is solitary work. But I also need and want to be out in the world. If

I didn't have this practice to come back to, I wouldn't have the rooting and the grounding that I need.

My practice used to be more strenuous and asana-based. In the last five to eight years, it's less so. Partly I'm trying to practice what I preach, which is "What are you feeling as you're doing these practices? How are they affecting you? How is it serving you? Is it serving you? Do you need to sit still? Do you need to move?" And I've had to surrender certain postures to the past.

Q. *As we grow older, then, our yoga practice may change? This is an interesting and I think important point.*

A. I wasn't in contact in the early years with many teachers who actually said, "As you get older you will benefit more by quieter forms of practice." My teachers were more about push, push, push. Fortunately I moved away from those teachers in time not to go on beating myself up for the fact that I couldn't continue as strenuous an asana practice as I had in earlier years.

It's not that I'm stiff by any means, or incapable — but I'm really listening to my body these days, and I find that my being needs to drink in that silent time of *pranayama* and meditation. That's where the nurturing is for me now. My practice is slower and quieter. Sometimes I will just sit for long periods of time or lie in a prone position. It's more spontaneous. It feels important to me now to sit still enough to let the difficulties of being alive arise and to face them, because I know that there are more coming.

What I discover as I age is that people don't just live a healthy life and then suddenly evaporate. Most of us are going to have to face a lot of slow time, and if we look at it as slow time as opposed to "Oh, this is a bummer: I can no longer do whatever," it can be a blessing. Whatever life brings us will continue to be a teaching and part of our practice. I think it's increasingly going to be important to help all of us make this shift in attitude.

Q. *Has this slowing down in your practice affected how you address other changes in your life?*

A. My father has ALS right now. He can't speak, but he can still write on his computer. I ask my mother, "Does he complain? Does he seem depressed? Does he seem angry?" "Oh, no, no, none of that," she answers. We had a family gathering recently, as we sometimes do, to cook together and laugh and talk and tell old stories. It gets raucous and loud and lots of laughter and my father just loves it. You can tell that he's just appreciating the family.

One day I was alone with him and I said to him, "Well, what do you think happens after we die?" He just looked at me — a longish kind of look — and then he shrugged his shoulders. He held that shrug for a few seconds, then let it go and went back to what he was doing. I realized he wasn't going to engage on this at all. I thought, "Oh God, he's just not willing to go there." Then I thought, "I wonder what that's about? Should I pursue this? Would it make sense? Could I have said it differently?"

I sat with it for the next couple of days, then I realized that he honestly — and who of us does? — doesn't know. And he's not going to speculate. He's not going to become suddenly a religious man in the very last months of his life. That's not what he goes for. In his own way he's spending a lot of time in meditation, reflection, or whatever. He's willing to be there, and he seems happy enough to be there. I realized that that is enough.

What I can take to him from my years of practice is simply the gift of presence in the face of this extremely heavy, sad time. It's been heartbreaking and heart opening and heart enlarging to be with him. I find that if I don't try to protect myself from the grief, it's so opening, so enlarging.

Q. *Who are the teachers who have inspired you?*

A. The inspiration from Yogananda was like an underground stream running through all my search for a path and a teacher, because of his intense desire to find a connection to spirit and to merge with what he called God. Much later the writings and life of Krishnamacharya became a powerful influence, because of his insatiable thirst for knowledge, his study of Ayurveda and languages, including Sanskrit, and his study of yoga in Tibet. I find there are so many sources of knowledge. Some teachers want us to limit ourselves to their way, but I've never been satisfied with that: I want to listen to all teachings and teachers and find out what works through the laboratory of my own body and life.

In terms of physical yoga practice, as I mentioned earlier, I started by practicing the yoga postures described in the books I was reading. Later I took classes with various teachers in Hawaii. But my study began more seriously when a close friend of mine and I began taking classes in San Francisco at what is now the Iyengar Yoga Institute. She was responsible for introducing me to Mr. Iyengar and his approach. I think the year was 1976. I recently saw again the video that had been made of him in 1976 in Ann Arbor, Michigan, and I realized why I was inspired by him. There was a masterful presence.

When I went to India to study with him, though, I had a very sad experience. He confronted me quite vehemently in front of other people. It was shocking to me — and an extremely shame-filled experience. Yet I was still inspired by him, and for the next ten to fifteen years I continued to follow that practice. I went to India two more times and took intensives with Mr. Iyengar's daughter, Geeta. But, looking back on it, I was never able to truly connect with him after that.

Q. *What was Mr. Iyengar confronting you about?*

A. Well, of course I was thirty-ish and young and headstrong. He was talking about doing yoga from the head, and I think he was probably saying something important, but the confrontation was so humiliating that I couldn't hear it. I will never treat someone like that. Some people have thrived under his teaching — obviously many people. I continue to be extremely grateful for his teaching. But not every teacher is meant for every student.

After that my relationship with teachers changed. There's a Zen teaching that says even the rocks and trees can be our teachers. I decided to take on the attitude that anyone I studied with could be a profound teacher for me. And in fact I think partly as a result of that attitude change, anyone I studied with *did* become a profound teacher for me. I think that adopting that view allowed me to keep a certain distance, which may or may not have been good. I never took on anyone as a guru. I just decided that every moment could be a dharma gate. There's a wonderful vow in Buddhism: "Dharma gates are boundless, I vow to enter them." That particular one of the four vows has always spoken to me very deeply.

Q. *Can you describe the vow in more detail?*

A. I think it's part of the *bodhisattva* vow. These may not be the only aspects of the vow, but the four that have meant much to me are:

> Beings are numberless; I vow to save them. Dharma gates are boundless; I vow to enter them. Illusions are inexhaustible; I vow to put an end to them. Buddha's ways are unsurpassable; I vow to become them.

When I heard "dharma gates are boundless" — being an artist I saw vistas everywhere I looked. If I let my gaze rest anywhere, there was a gate and it was beckoning me. It's a wonderful vision of possibility. If only we allow ourselves to walk through those gates, I truly believe that all of life becomes our teacher. ●

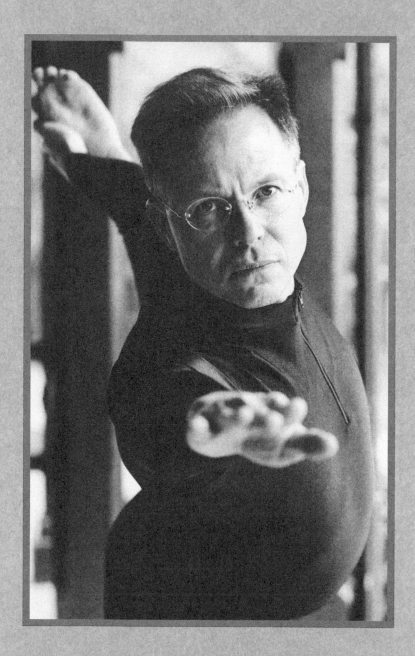

Stephen Cope

EVERYTHING IS ALREADY OK

STEPHEN COPE is a psychotherapist, yoga teacher, and author. In 1989 he left his psychotherapy practice in Boston to spend a year's sabbatical at Kripalu Center for Yoga & Health — then one of the largest ashrams in America. After that year, he decided to become part of the community. Only five years later Kripalu's longtime spiritual director resigned, and Stephen was one of a group of students who stayed on to rebuild the community into a thriving nonprofit educational center for contemplative practice and study. Today he savors being part of a post-guru community in which the wisdom of a two-thousand-year-old tradition inheres in the community as a whole rather than in one charismatic leader. Stephen's book, *Yoga and the Quest for the True Self*, was published in 1999, an autobiographical account of a Western seeker exploring the psychology of yoga. • Stephen traces his passion for hatha yoga back to an early career in dance. He was one of the first students at Amherst College to participate in the dance departments at Smith and Mount Holyoke Colleges, and went on to dance professionally for a regional ballet and modern-dance company. He was thrilled at midlife to discover yoga as a way to keep dance in his life, and he has been particularly drawn to Kripalu yoga for its flowing, meditative, and dancelike style.

EVEN AS A YOUNG BOY I was fascinated by spirituality. I loved going to church — though I didn't let it be widely known, since I was only marginally passing as "cool" anyway. I was stirred by the ecstatic Bach chorales sung by the choir in the small Presbyterian college chapel where my family worshipped every Sunday. After church I would secretly learn the chorales on the piano and sing them to myself. They had exotic German names: *Wachet Auf!* Sleepers, Wake! I felt strangely at home with the stately processions, the archaic language of scripture, the sense of the numinous. And — go figure — I was actually interested in the long and sometimes theologically tedious sermons. My father and I would argue about them at Sunday dinner — over a table laden with roast beef and green bean casserole — while the rest of the family rolled their eyes in boredom.

At eighteen I decamped from the cornfields of central Ohio to the ivy-covered halls of a New England college and eventually on to Boston for graduate school. When I arrived at a well-known Boston-area psychiatric hospital for my first graduate clinical training placement, I discovered that one of my supervisors was none other than my former Christian Youth Fellowship Director from back home. Egad! He had become so urbane: Not only was he training to become a psychologist, but he had already become a Buddhist. One afternoon I went with him to sit at the local meditation center. We meditated together for an hour. Nothing has really been the same since.

"There is room for all of you in this practice," he said. "No part of you has to go into exile." That sounded good. I began to meditate. I stopped by the meditation center every evening on my way home from graduate school, and spent all day Sunday sitting and walking, sitting and walking (two different forms of meditation). When I emerged from these Sunday daylong sits, the world looked transformed. Everything was bathed in light. Colors vibrated with intensity. And everything was incontrovertibly OK. Just absolutely OK. Sometimes I cried all the way home, averting my gaze from onlookers in passing cars. "What's wrong?" my partner, David, would ask when I arrived home red-eyed. "I don't know," I'd say. "I'm happy."

> "Finally I had found a tradition
> that understood the days to be gods!
> The moments to be gods!"

My early experiences with meditation were ecstatic. Christian monastics call these ecstatic experiences "the consolations of the spiritual life." Buddhists say their nature is *sukkha:* sweetness. For whatever reasons, early on in my meditation practice I had a great deal of sweetness. I discovered that when I was not craving and clinging for some other experience, I was just happy. Happy with Being itself! Who knew?

Soon I began to read the burgeoning contemplative literature: Chogyam Trungpa, Rinpoche; Suzuki Roshi; Achaan Chah. I was blown away by the sheer intellectual and psychological brilliance of Buddhism. Here was a real path — a spiritual ascent that actually offered a detailed *practice.* In my spiritual life so far, there had been plenty of theology but virtually no instruction in practice. How do you meditate? How do you pray? How do you know God? In the traditions of my childhood, it was all so ineffable. I guess one was supposed to work it out between oneself and God. In Buddhism I discovered an astonishingly systematic — almost scientific — "technique." I found that very helpful.

I was thrilled, too, to discover that the Buddha taught that our problems are not metaphysical, not "theological," but existential. I had intuited this all along: It's not *what you know* that counts. It's *how you live*. How you live every day. In college I had been deeply devoted to Emerson and Thoreau, and knew Emerson was right when he said that every day is the day of creation and the day of judgment. "Heaven," he said, "walks among us ordinarily muffled in such triple or tenfold disguises that the wisest are deceived and no one suspects the days to be gods." (*Emerson: The Mind on Fire;* Robert D. Richardson, Jr., University of California Press, 1995, p. 342)

Finally I had found a tradition that understood the days to be gods! The moments to be gods! The magic and practical wisdom of the contemplative traditions drew me in rather quickly. I began to sit long retreats. Before long I was on fire with the Dharma.

All of that was almost thirty years ago. Wow! That went fast. Now my life is thoroughly organized around the contemplative traditions — both yoga and Buddhism. (Twelve years after I discovered Buddhism, I found yoga and, inevitably, Kripalu.) It's fun to think back, now, on those early years of discovery. And it's fun to ponder the question that I've posed for so many of my friends in this volume. Have yoga and meditation really changed my life?

For me, I guess the answer has to be both yes and no.

* * *

The older I get, the more I realize that I am exactly the way I was at thirteen — that kid singing the Bach chorales. I'm still exactly like that. This realization is full of irony, because I've spent so much of my life trying to change myself. I was such a neurotic twenty- and thirtysomething. Always striving — always trying to live up to some ideal notion of who I *should* be. I was deeply affected by the culture of my elite New England college (Amherst), where most of us were striving so hard to be Somebody in the world. Most of my friends, of course, already *were* Somebody — or so it appeared to me. As a hayseed from Ohio, I had a lot of catching up to do. And I worked very hard at it. Always the overachiever. But, of course, the harder I worked, the less satisfied I was. The problem, I learned later, was, well . . . that I *wasn't* anyone.

At fifty I can say that the only thing that has really changed is that I have begun to accept who I already am. The gift of con- templative practice for me has been radical self-acceptance. I've begun to learn to make room for both the *neuroses* and the *magnifi- cence,* such as they are. (And I think there's some of each.) What makes this possible is that I can now view them as "the neuroses" and "the magnificence." They're not really "mine." It's all so much more impersonal than I thought: just causes and conditions, playing themselves out and passing away (karma). What a relief. This means

that I don't have to remain overidentified with "my" story —
which, of course, like all of our stories, gets boring pretty fast.

Has practice changed my life? Well, I can say with certainty
that it's changed where I stand in relationship to the whole drama of
life. Through practice I've come to see that the deepest source of my
misery is not wanting things to be the way they are. Not wanting
myself to be the way I am. Not wanting the world to be the way it
is. Not wanting others to be the way they are. Whenever I'm suffering, I find this "war with reality" to be at the heart of the problem.

My entire practice — both yoga and meditation — is about
learning to be present with "the way it is." This is an easier way to
live in the world than the way of striving and clinging and craving.
The great Thai forest master Achaan Chah has been perhaps my
central teacher in this practice. From the moment I first read his
words in Jack Kornfield's *A Still Forest Pool,* I was taken by his simplicity, directness, and intellectual precision.

> Try to do everything with a mind that lets go.
> If you let go a little you will have a little peace.
> If you let go a lot, you will have a lot of peace.
> If you let go completely, you will know complete
>   peace and freedom.
> Your struggles with the world will have come
>   to an end.

That is really the heart of my practice. I'm pretty sure that the
most important thing I've learned is this: I can entrust myself, and
my life, to the natural intelligence of a still and radiant mind — the

mind that lets go. When the mind is quiet, all wisdom reveals itself effortlessly. All I have to do is stay tuned. In order to do that, I constantly need to slow down the drama. As Don Juan said to his student Carlos Castaneda: "You must learn to stop the world!" When I'm speeding through life, it usually means that I'm on automatic pilot — acting out my conditioned patterns (samsaras). For me, that means charging ahead with my big plans and schemes to be Someone, to achieve this or that, or to get this or that. No matter how many years I practice, this tendency to want to be Somebody remains strong.

I've found, however, that practice cuts through that tendency more quickly these days. I've learned to trust what I call "the braille method" of living — relinquishing grand plans and schemes in favor of an intuitive approach, feeling my way from tree to tree, relinquishing my attempts to control the world and learning, instead, to trust a discerning surrender. My best friend, Adam, puts this so well. When confronted with a conundrum he says, "Well. Let life do it." Exactly. Willpower is the caveman approach to life.

Finally, I'm learning to live inside the view (central to both yoga and Buddhism) that everything is really already OK. I may not understand it, but I know that it's so. And this allows me to relax my grip on life. With age I'm even learning to relax my grip on practice. This is because I see more and more irrevocably that *what I am hunting is also hunting for me.* I do not have to be "the Doer."

Living as "not the Doer" is a surprising way to live. I never know what's going to happen. I'm no longer living with the illusion of control. It's exciting. And it can be very passionate. The great irony is that the less I "do," the more gets "done." The less I try to be Somebody, the more somebody appears, moment to moment. Classes get taught, my house gets cleaned, articles get written, dinners with friends get organized. Who's doing it all? I don't know. Not I.

> "I've learned to trust what I call 'the braille method' of living — relinquishing grand plans and schemes in favor of an intuitive approach, feeling my way from tree to tree."

Franz Kafka said it so very well: "Become still and quiet inside and the world will roll at your feet. It has no choice." The most wonderful fruit of practice for me is a growing delight with Being itself — a delight I seem to have known intensely as a kid, but which I've had to relearn as an adult. Yoga and meditation have helped me so much. Sleepers, Wake! •

Glossary

NOTE: Literal meanings are included in quotation marks.

ACHAAN (also spelled **AJAHN** and **AJAAN**). Buddhist term for an influential teacher or mentor.

ADVAITA. "Nondual." A school of Vedanta having its roots in the *Upanishads* that teaches that reality is not split between subject and object, but one reality expressed in the form of absolute consciousness.

AJAHN (also spelled **AJAAN** and **ACHAAN**). Buddhist term for an influential teacher or mentor.

ANAPANASATI. Mindfulness of breath; a meditation practice in which attention is focused on the breath as a way to calm the mind.

ANATTA. Nonexistence of self, in which the ego is seen as transitory and changing rather than permanent or eternal.

ANICCA. Impermanence or transitoriness; refers to all things in the phenomenal world that arise, dwell, and pass away.

ANUSARA YOGA. Yoga style developed by John Friend in 1997 that couples precise alignment in hatha yoga postures with Tantric philosophy. The word *Anusara* means "flowing with grace."

ARTI (also spelled **ARATI**). An offering of light, usually in the form of a camphor or ghee lamp, made to a deity or guru and generally accompanied by a devotional song or prayer.

ASANA. "Seat." Usually refers to any of the various hatha yoga postures. The third limb of Patanjali's eight limbs of yoga.

ASHRAM. A hermitage or sanctuary where students study and practice the teachings of a guru, or spiritual teacher.

ASHTANGA. Eight-limbed path of yoga articulated by Patanjali; Ashtanga yoga can also refer to a contemporary form of hatha yoga characterized by an intensive *vinyasa* practice.

AUTOBIOGRAPHY OF A YOGI. A spiritual classic written by Paramahansa Yogananda in 1946 about his life in India. The book served as an inspirational and exotic introduction to the traditions of yoga and meditation for many spiritual seekers.

AVATAR. Manifestation or incarnation of the divine on earth.

AYURVEDA. "Life Science." A traditional Indian healing system dating back to 4000 BCE that emphasizes the harmony of the whole being.

BHAGHAVAD-GITA. "Song of the Lord." Part of the epic Indian poem *The Mahabharata*, the *Gita* is a dialogue between the warrior Arjuna and his charioteer, Lord Krishna, about the deeper teachings of yoga. It is believed to have been written around 200 BCE.

BHAKTA. A person who follows the path of devotion and practices love for and surrender to God.

BHAKTI. "Devotion." Love of God; surrender to the divine.

BODHISATTVA. "Enlightened Being." Usually refers to a person who has committed his or her life to the liberation of all beings.

BRAHMACHARI. Usually refers to a monk or nun; one who has taken vows of chastity and lives according to strict rules of conduct and moral discipline.

BRAHMAN. The eternal, absolute, nondual ground of being in Vedanta (not to be confused with Brahma, the creator god of the Hindu trinity).

BUDDHISM. Religious and philosophical tradition of practice and thought that arose from the teachings of Siddhartha Gautama in India around 500 BCE and spread, in various forms, throughout the world.

CHAKRA. "Wheel, Circle." Center of subtle, concentrated energy in the body. Most systems refer to seven such centers, aligned along the midpoint of the body from the base of the spine to the crown of the head.

CITTA. Mind, heart, consciousness, cognition, attentiveness.

DHARMA. In Buddhism, *dharma* refers to the teachings of the Buddha. In general usage it refers to the way or path, a way of life leading to ultimate reality; it is often used to mean one's particular life mission.

DIAMOND SUTRA. Part of the Buddhist *Prajnaparamita Sutra*, teaching that appearances in the phenomenal world are not ultimate reality, but rather projections of the mind.

DITTHI. Clinging to views; right or wrong view.

DUKKHA. Suffering, dissatisfaction, incompleteness, pain, distress, discontent; a central concept in Buddhism referring not just to unpleasant sensations or experiences, but rather to anything in the material and mental realms that is impermanent.

DZOGCHEN. "Great Perfection," a primary teaching of one school of Tibetan Buddhism that holds that the mind is naturally pure, and needs only to be recognized and experienced as such.

EIGHT LIMBS OF YOGA. A path to superconsciousness as codified in Patanjali's *Yoga-Sutra*. The path includes: 1. *yamas* (behaviors to avoid); 2. *niyamas* (ethical practices); 3. asanas (physical positions or postures of the body); 4. *pranayama* (breath control); 5. *pratyahara* (withdrawal of the senses; 6. *dharana* (concentration); 7. *dhyana* (meditation); 8. *samadhi* (ecstasy).

EIGHTFOLD PATH OF BUDDHA. Path to end suffering taught by the Buddha; right view, right intention, right speech, right action, right livelihood, right effort, right mindfulness, right concentration.

ENLIGHTENMENT. English word for the Sanskrit term *bodhi,* or awakened; attainment of truth, liberation, or self-realization, where the limited sense of "I" merges into supreme consciousness.

FREEMASONRY. International movement whose members work for charitable and social causes and practice secret rituals. Thirteen U.S. presidents have been Masons.

GANESHA. Elephant-headed deity; son of Shiva and Parvati; remover of obstacles said to give wisdom and success in both the worldly and the spiritual realms.

GENJOKOAN. "Enlightenment Appears in Everyday Life." A chapter from the Japanese Zen master Dogen's *Shobo-genzo* that discusses the connection between Zen practice and enlightenment.

GESTALT THERAPY. School of psychology founded by Fritz Perls in the 1940s that emphasizes the patient's here/now experience and behavior, as well as the use of focused awareness and experimentation to achieve insight.

GNOSTIC. A segment of the early (fourth-century) Christian Church that believed that knowledge is acquired by direct experience, and that personal knowledge of truth is accessible to all.

GURU. Hindu term for teacher, spiritual master, guide, or adviser; often said to be one who dispels darkness or leads the disciple from darkness into light.

HASIDIC. Branch of Orthodox Judaism founded by Ba'al Shem Tov in 1734, distinguished by its focus on mystical insight and feeling the presence of God in all aspects of life.

HATHA YOGA. The physical system of control of the body utilizing asana (postures) and *pranayama* (regulation of the breath). *Ha* means sun, *Tha* means moon; hatha yoga is said to achieve balance by combining opposing forces.

HATHAYOGA-PRADIPIKA. Classic work on hatha yoga consisting of 395 verses written by Svatmarama in the 16th century.

HEART SUTRA. The shortest of the 40 sutras that make up the *Prajnaparamita Sutra* of Buddhism. It is known for the pithy declaration: "Form is no other than emptiness; emptiness is no other than form."

INTEGRAL YOGA. Contemporary school of yoga based on the teachings of Swami Satchidananda, in the lineage of Swami Sivananada of Rishikesh.

ISHVARA PRANIDHANA. "Surrender to God." This is one of the *niyamas* in Patanjali's second limb of yoga, and requires dedicating all efforts and activities to God.

IYENGAR YOGA. Contemporary school of yoga created by B.K.S. Iyengar in the lineage of Krishnamacharya, which encourages precise alignment and attention to the physical details of postures.

JIVA. "Living or Existing Being." Generally signifies the finite, biological personality or psyche; the mortal, embodied self bound to the cycle of birth and death.

JNANA YOGA. "Yoga of Wisdom." Going to God through discrimination, knowledge, questioning, and contemplation.

JUKAI. "Receiving the Precepts." The ceremonial initiation into Buddhism through receiving and acknowledging the Buddhist precepts.

KAGYU SECT. Tibetan Buddhist lineage that traces back to Marpa, Naropa, and Milarepa and teaches Mahamudra, the Tantric practices of the tradition. One branch of the sect is headed by the Karmapa.

KAMMATTHANA. A Buddhist Thai forest tradition founded by Phra Ajaan Mun and Phra Ajaan Sao.

KARMA. "Action or Deed." Volitional act that results in reward or retribution in this or future lifetimes; destiny or fate; the cosmic law of cause and effect.

KARMAPA. The spiritual head of the Kagyu school of Tibetan Buddhism. There have been 17 incarnations of the Karmapa since the 12th century.

KASHMIR SHAIVISM. Branch of Tantric Shaivism (Shiva worship) that emerged in Kashmir between 700 and 1100 CE; a nondual tradition that holds that the world is absolute consciousness.

KOAN. A paradoxical phrase or teaching on Zen realization, often posed as a question for students to work with. Koans can't be answered by using reason, but only by transcending the limitation of thought or logic, making an intuitive leap to a different state of consciousness.

KRIPALU YOGA. Contemporary style of yoga originated by Yogi Amrit Desai and further developed by his Western disciples. It is named for Yogi Desai's guru, Swami Kripalu, and emphasizes the practices of being present in the body and witness consciousness.

KRIYAVATI. Spontaneous hatha yoga postures arising from awakened kundalini; a state where a practitioner flows into even the most difficult yoga postures without effort.

KUNDALINI. "Coiled One, or Snake." Known as the serpent power, this dormant spiritual energy is said to lie coiled at the base of the spine. Once aroused, the energy moves upward through the chakras and results in spiritual awakening.

KUNDALINI YOGA. Contemporary school of yoga created by Yogi Bhajan and taught by the 3HO organization; more broadly, any yoga aimed at awakening the latent power of kundalini energy.

LAMA. Tibetan Buddhist spiritual teacher or mentor, a guide on the path to enlightenment; one who is qualified to perform Tantric rituals.

LIGHT ON YOGA. Classic book by B.K.S. Iyengar published in 1966; a handbook of hatha yoga containing more than 600 illustrations and showing details of over 200 postures and other yogic practices.

LOVINGKINDNESS. The English word for *metta,* the Buddhist meditation practice that cultivates caring and compassion for oneself and others.

MAHAMUDRA. "Great Seal." One of the highest teachings of the Kagyu sect of Tibetan Buddhism leading to spiritual freedom through realization of emptiness *(shunyata)* and freedom from death and rebirth (samsara).

MAHAYANA. "Great Vehicle." One of the two great schools of Buddhism (the other is Hinayana) that arose in the first century CE. Mahayana stresses not just the liberation of the individual, but also seeking to attain enlightenment for the sake of all beings, and looks to the teachings of the Buddha and his tradition of enlightened masters.

MAITRI. "Kindness, Benevolence." Refers to the Tibetan Buddhist practice of lovingkindness, or benevolence toward all beings.

MANTRA. A sacred sound that can be a syllable or series of syllables, or a name for God. Repetition of a mantra is said to help concentrate and clear the mind and even lead to God-realization.

MARA. Buddhist "tempter" figure who tries to divert right action or pose hindrances to enlightenment. Mara can be interpreted as a real person or as a metaphor for greed, hatred, and delusion.

MEDITATION. General term given to a host of different practices that help focus the mind so the practitioner can reach a state of awakening or liberation.

METTA. "Lovingkindness, goodwill." A meditation practice that directs a prayer of well-being toward oneself and/or others.

MIDDLE PATH. The way of the historical Buddha, who taught moderation, and the avoidance of all extremes.

MINDFULNESS. Performing all activities consciously, even routine actions like breathing and walking.

MINDFULNESS MEDITATION. Often used as a synonym for Vipassana, this practice involves the moment-to-moment awareness of all aspects of daily life, witnessing what is in the mind without reaction or involvement.

MOKSHA. "Liberation." Release from the cycle of birth and death.

NADA. "Sound." The primal vibration, manifesting as inner, mystical sound.

NADI SHODHANA. "Purification of the Channels." An alternate-nostril breathing technique said to calm the mind, purify the nerves, and open the energy channels.

NAMA. "Name." Conditioned reality; the many names by which the divine is worshipped.

NIYAMA. "Minor Restraint." Five disciplines or observances set out in the *Yoga-Sutra* of Patanjali as the second of his eight limbs of yoga. Consists of the practices of purity, contentment, austerity, study of sacred texts, and devotion or surrender to God.

NOBLE TRUTHS. The four essential teachings of Buddhism: Existence is characterized by suffering; suffering is caused by craving; suffering can be ended by eliminating craving; this can be achieved by following the eightfold path.

OM. Primordial sound vibration regarded as the seed of all mantras; a one-syllable mantra expressing the oneness of the universe.

PARAMATMAN. "Supreme Self." The transcendent, universal self or consciousness.

PITI. "Rapture." Bliss, happiness, delight; any of a number of qualities of mind or heightened energy states in the body experienced in meditation.

PRAJNA. "Wisdom." In Buddhism, an experience of intuitive wisdom or insight that cannot be conveyed by intellectual concepts.

PRANA. "Life, or Breath of Life." The life force or energy that sustains the body and distinguishes the animate from the inanimate, most noticeable as breath.

PRANAYAMA. "Breath Control." A variety of exercises aimed at controlling the breath and energizing the body; the fourth of Patanjali's eight limbs.

PRATYAHARA. "Withdrawal." Sensory withdrawal or inhibition; a state of introversion attained by internalizing the senses; the fifth of Patanjali's eight limbs.

PREM. Divine, spiritual, or pure love.

PUJA. "Worship or Adoration." Acts of reverence performed to some aspect of the divine, such as offering flowers or fruit to a deity.

PUNDIT. A learned or wise person or scholar; a term of respect for a person of knowledge; can also refer to a Hindu priest.

PURE YOGA. Contemporary yoga school developed by Rod Stryker that is a synthesis of yoga postures, Tantric philosophy, meditation, and breathing practices, with the aim of mastering the life force in the body.

QIGONG. A key component in traditional Chinese medicine with a history going back nearly 5,000 years, this self-healing art combines movement, meditation, and relaxation, working with life energy in the body.

RAJA YOGA. "Royal Yoga." Another name for Patanjali's eight limbs of yoga, aimed at purifying body and mind to lead the practitioner to enlightenment.

ROLFING. System of structural integration named for developer Dr. Ida P. Rolf. Rolfing utilizes soft tissue manipulation, particularly with the myofascial system (connective tissues), and is said to align and balance the body.

RUPA. "Form." Can refer to the body, physical beauty, the visible or manifest world.

SADHANA. "Realizing or to Arrive at the Goal." Systematic spiritual practice or discipline intended to transform body and mind; the path of spiritual realization.

SADHUS. Holy persons, often monks, who have renounced the world and wander from place to place seeking to realize God.

SAKSHIN. "Witness." The observer, or witness consciousness; another name for the transcendental Self.

SAMADHI. In Buddhism, the word is translated as "Concentration" and refers to a focused state of mind free from distraction. In yoga this word is translated as "Ecstasy" and refers to a state of superconsciousness in which total absorption in the object of meditation has been achieved, and the ego disappears.

SAMSARA. "Journeying." The cycle of birth, death, and rebirth; the finite, changing world.

SAMSKARAS. "Impressions." Tendencies or patterns that have arisen through actions and thoughts in this or earlier births, and which enmesh us in the world of change.

SANGHA. In Buddhism, refers to the Buddhist community of practitioners; more broadly, any group of seekers who gather to realize truth.

SATORI. Zen term for the experience of awakening or enlightenment; a flash of awareness or realization.

SAVASANA. Hatha yoga posture; Corpse Pose, the pose of deep relaxation.

SESSHIN. Retreat for Zen practitioners; days of especially focused, intensive meditation practice.

SEVA. "Service." Selfless service; service done with an attitude of deep devotion and without attachment to the fruits of the labor.

SHABD. "Sound." The sound of God; the essence of all things.

SHAKTI. "Power, Force, or Energy." Divine power or primal energy; in Hinduism, Shakti is personified as the consort of Shiva, the female, dynamic, creative force in the universe.

SHAMATHA (also spelled **SAMATHA**). "Dwelling in Tranquillity." A meditation technique that calms the mind and heightens concentration.

SHANTI. "Peace." Calm, spiritual peace, mental equilibrium.

SHIVA. Third deity in the Hindu trinity, who functions as the god of transformation and destruction. He is seen as the destroyer of ignorance and worldliness and the originator of yoga.

SHRI (also spelled **SRI**). "Beauty, Majesty, Blessed, Holy." In this context, shri refers to the quality of divine beauty in the form.

SHUNYATA (also spelled **SUNYATA**). "Emptiness." Central tenet of Buddhism that holds that all phenomenal things are empty and impermanent. This doesn't mean the phenomenal world doesn't exist, but rather that it is devoid of essence; it is there in appearance only.

SIDDHIS. "Accomplishments." Supernatural abilities appearing as by-products of spiritual development. These powers can include the ability to read minds, levitate, enter other bodies, and become invisible.

SIKH. "Disciple." Spiritual tradition for householders founded by Guru Nanak (1469–1539 CE) in India, and based upon the teachings of ten Sikh gurus, the last of whom was Guru Gobind Singh (1666–1708 CE).

SILA (also spelled **SHILA**). Virtue or morality; the practices or precepts that keep one from unskillful acts; the rules of ethical conduct and discipline established by the Buddha.

SO HAM. "He am I." One of the mantras of nondual Vedanta that identifies the individual self with the universal self.

SRI VIDYA. "Blessed Knowledge." An esoteric, Tantric tradition dating back to the 10th or 11th century in south India, related to Kashmir Shaivism's nondual teachings.

STHIRA SUKHA. "Steady comfort." Patanjali's instruction for yoga postures; stability and feeling of well-being resulting from doing asanas; a steady, comfortable sitting posture for meditation.

STUPA. "Hair Knot." Buddhist architecture with tall, spired monuments and temples. Originally built over mortal remains or relics of saints, now stupas often serve as symbolic reminders of the awakened state.

SUFI. A follower of the mystical, esoteric path of Islam that rose as an organized movement between 660 and 750 AD. Sufis seek direct personal experience of God, and believe it is possible to experience intimacy with God while alive.

SUKKHA (also spelled **SUKHA**). "Joy, Pleasure, Ease." Sweetness, happiness, bliss, satisfaction; a mental quality of meditation.

SURAT SHABD YOGA. Practice whose object is to attune to the current of sound or spiritual current always vibrating within, involving meditation on inner sound and light.

SUTRA. "Thread." In yoga, sutras are pithy teachings, often accompanied by commentaries, such as Patanjali's *Yoga-Sutra*. In Buddhism sutras refer to the discourses of the Buddha.

SVAROOPA YOGA. Contemporary school of yoga developed by Rama Berch and sometimes referred to as "Bliss Yoga," which emphasizes inner experience through the practice of postures using both compassion and precision.

SWAMI. Term of respect or honorific used for a monk who has vowed to renounce worldly life; title of a Hindu monk belonging to a monastic order.

TAI CHI. Form of Chinese martial art dating back to the 13th century CE, often practiced for its health benefits; a form of moving meditation, characterized by slow, flowing movements.

TANTRA. "Loom, Continuum." A Hindu and Buddhist movement that teaches the underlying unity of spirit and matter and emphasizes that a worldly life is not an impediment to spiritual awakening.

TANTRIKA. One who practices Tantra.

TAOISM. Chinese philosophy/religion/way of life founded by Lao Tzu (604–531 BCE) and based on his book, the *Tao Te Ching*. The Tao is the way, or path, or the force that flows through all things. Taoism stresses the balance of opposites.

TEJAS. "Brilliance." The light that radiates from a saint, said to be the result of intense spiritual practices or asceticism.

THEOSOPHY. "Divine Wisdom." A synthesis of science, religion, and philosophy based on the direct and immediate experience of the divine, started by H.P. Blavatsky and H.S. Olcott in 1875 to promulgate divine truth.

THERAVADAN BUDDHISM (also spelled **THERAVADIN**). A school of Buddhism focusing exclusively on the Buddha's teachings, versus later enlightened beings, now widespread in Thailand, Burma, Sri Lanka, Cambodia, and Laos, in which emphasis is placed on liberation of the individual through meditation and observance of moral disciplines.

3HO FOUNDATION. Happy, Healthy, Holy Organization, founded by Yogi Bhajan in 1969. It operates more than 300 centers in 35 countries.

TIBETAN BUDDHISM. Form of Mahayana Buddhism practiced not only in Tibet, but also in the neighboring countries of the Himalayas. It has been described as a blend of Buddhism, Indian Tantric practices, and Tibetan shamanism.

UJJAYI. "Victorious, Victory." Often called the Ocean Sounding breath; performed by slightly constricting the back of the throat to create an audible breathing sound, used as an aid in focusing the mind.

UPANISHADS. "Sitting Close to One's Teacher." A collection of Hindu scriptures that make up the final portion of the *Vedas* and contain esoteric, nondual teachings believed to have been composed between 700 and 300 BCE.

UPAVISTA KONASANA. Hatha yoga posture known as the Seated Angle or Wide Angle Pose.

UPAYA. "Means." Skill in means or methods, such as those used by the Buddha in teaching his students in accordance with their capabilities.

UTTHITA PARSVAKONASANA. Hatha yoga posture known as the Extended Side Angle Pose or the Extended Lateral Angle.

VAJRASANA. Hatha yoga posture known as the Thunderbolt Pose, sitting with the buttocks on the heels.

VEDANA. "Feeling, Sensation." The Buddhist term for all feelings, which can be categorized as pleasant, unpleasant, or neutral.

VEDANTA. One of the classical philosophies of Hinduism; the conclusion of the *Vedas*, including the *Upanishads*, expounding that the universe is derived from a single essence called Brahman; the cornerstone of present-day Hinduism.

VEDAS. "Knowledge, Sacred Teachings." The oldest texts of Hindu literature; the sacred knowledge contained in four collections, collectively known as the *Vedas*.

VEGAN. Strictest form of vegetarianism, whose adherents eat no animal products and avoid leather, fur, wool, and cosmetics tested on animals.

VINIYOGA. Contemporary school of yoga developed by T. Krishnamacharya and his son T.K.V. Desikachar that encourages adaptations to each student's unique physical needs and emphasizes linking breath with movement.

VINYASA. "Connecting." Style of yoga in which postures are performed in a connected, flowing fashion, synchronized with breath.

VIPASSANA. Often used in the West to refer to a technique of insight meditation; in Mahayana Buddhism, refers to the examination of the nature of things, leading to clear insight into the impermanence of physical and mental phenomena.

VISHUDIMAGGA (also spelled **VISUDDHI-MAGGA**). "Path of Purity." An important writing in Theravadan Buddhism composed in the fifth century by Buddhaghosha, dealing with moral discipline, meditation, and wisdom.

WICCA. Nature-oriented pagan religion with practices to align with natural rhythms and find balance within self and universe.

WU-MEN-KWAN. "Gateless Gate." One of the two most important koan collections in Zen literature, compiled in China in the 13th century. It consists of 48 koans, each with a brief commentary, and was written by the Chinese Zen master Wu-men Hui-k'ai.

YAMA. "Restraint." First of Patanjali's eight limbs of yoga, made up of five restraints or moral precepts: nonviolence, non-lying, non-stealing, moderation in all things, and non-possessiveness.

YOGA. "Union or Yoke." A large and varied body of spiritual and mystical practices that arose in India as far back as 5,000 years ago as a way to achieve union with the divine; in the West, yoga usually refers to hatha yoga, or physical postures and breathing exercises.

YOGA NIDRA. Yogic "sleep" in which the body is relaxed while the mind remains fully conscious; deep relaxation typically practiced at the end of a hatha yoga session.

YOGA-SUTRA. A collection of 195 aphorisms written by Patanjali in the second century BCE, considered to be the primary text of classical yoga.

YOGA, YOUTH & REINCARNATION. Book by Jess Stearn published in 1965 and considered by many to be a metaphysical classic.

YOGI. One who practices yoga; a title signifying an accomplished male practitioner of yoga.

YOGIN. Male yoga practitioner.

YOGINI. Female yoga practitioner.

ZEN. A school of Mahayana Buddhism that arose in China in the sixth and seventh centuries that stresses the importance of practice and direct experience for the attainment of liberation.

Key Teachers
(As Mentioned in Text)

ACHAAN. *see* **CHAH.**

AJAHN. *see* **SUMEDHO** and **SUWAT.**

AJAYA, SWAMI (1940–   ). Born Allan Weinstock, he trained as a clinical psychologist before being ordained a monk in the order of Shankaracharya by his guru, Swami Rama, at the Himalayan Institute, Honesdale, PA. His books include *Psychotherapy East and West: A Unifying Paradigm* (1983) and *Yoga Psychology* (1974).

AMBIKANANDA SARASWATI, SWAMI. A Hindu monk who teaches yoga and Vedanta philosophy in England, she is a qualified practitioner of Chinese medicine and founder of the Traditional Yoga Association, based in the U.K. She is a student of Swami Venkatesananda and was initiated by Swami Chidananda. Her books include *Katha Upanishad* (2001) and *Healing Yoga* (2001).

BADARAYANA. A teacher with experience in both the yoga and Buddhist traditions, he requested that his identity not be revealed.

BALASKAS, ARTHUR. Yoga teacher, associate of R.D. Laing, he was also active in the breathwork movement. Author of *Bodylife* (1977).

BALSEKAR, RAMESH S. Advaita master living in Bombay, India, whose key teaching is "All that is, is Consciousness," he was a student of Nisargadatta Maharaj. Author of *Consciousness Speaks: Conversations With Ramesh S. Balsekar,* edited by Wayne Liquorman (1992).

BAPTISTE, MAGANA. A student of Yogananda, yoga teacher, and dancer, she founded the first school of Middle Eastern dance in San Francisco. With her husband, Walt, she opened one of the first yoga studios in San Francisco in 1955. She is the author of *Breath Is Life* (1980).

BHAJAN, YOGI (1929–   ). Founder of 3HO (the Healthy, Happy, Holy Organization) and spiritual head of the Sikh Dharma of the Western Hemisphere, he came to the U.S. in 1968 and began teaching kundalini yoga and meditation and sharing Sikh teachings. Author of *Teachings of Yogi Bhajan* (1977) and other titles.

BOWMAN, GEORGE. Founder of Institute for the Study of Meditation and Psychotherapy in Cambridge, MA, he was a student of Seung Sahn and Joshu Sasaki. He currently lives at Furnace Mountain Zen Center in Kentucky.

THE BUDDHA (dates vary, usually sixth century BCE). Born Siddhartha Gautama in northern India, he achieved enlightenment at age 35 after years of asceticism and seeking, then spent the next 45 years teaching the path he called the "Middle Way." The title "Buddha" is given to an enlightened one, or one who rediscovers the path of dharma.

CASTANEDA, CARLOS (1931–1998). Anthropologist known for a series of books about his spiritual training with a Mexican shaman named Don Juan. He was born in Peru and became an American citizen in 1959. His books include *The Teachings of Don Juan: A Yaqui Way of Knowledge* (1968).

CHAH, ACHAAN (ca.1917–1992). Thai forest meditation master who lived in the monastery of Wat Ba Pong; teacher of Jack Kornfield and other Western Vipassana teachers; author of *A Still Forest Pool*, edited by Jack Kornfield (1985), and *Food for the Heart: The Collected Teachings of Ajahn Chah* (2002).

CHETANANANDA, SWAMI. American meditation master and abbot of Nityananda Institute, he trained under Swami Rudrananda and embraced Kashmiri Shaivism, using kundalini yoga as the vehicle for realization.

CHIDANANDA, SWAMI (1916–   ). President of the Divine Life Society in Rishikesh, India; born Sridhar Rao in south India, he is a disciple of Swami Sivananda of Rishikesh. He became president of the Divine Life Society when Swami Sivananda died in 1963. Author of *Awake! Realize Your Divinity* (1999) and *A New Beginning* (1991).

CHIDVILASANANDA, GURUMAYI. Successor to Swami Muktananda, she is the head of the SYDA Foundation and author of numerous books and recordings, including *Courage and Contentment: A Collection of Talks on Spiritual Life* (1999).

CHINO, KOBUN (1938–2002). Zen master, calligrapher, poet, and painter who came to the U.S. from Japan in 1967 and helped establish Tassajara monastery with Shunryu Suzuki Roshi. He was teaching at Naropa Institute at the time of his death.

CHOUDHURY, BIKRAM (1946–). Founded Bikram's Yoga College of India in California in 1974. Born in Calcutta, he studied yoga with Bishnu Ghosh, brother of Paramahansa Yogananda, and designed a 26-asana series, done in a specific order in a heated room, popularly known as Bikram's yoga. Author of *Bikram's Beginning Yoga Class* (1978).

DALAI LAMA (1935–). Born Tenzin Gyatso in Tibet, he was deemed the reincarnation of the Dalai Lama at age two. Recognized as the spiritual and temporal leader of the Tibetan people, he fled Tibet in 1959 and settled in Dharamsala, India. He won the Nobel Peace Prize in 1989 and is the author of many books, including *Freedom in Exile: The Autobiography of the Dalai Lama* (1990).

DESAI, YOGI AMRIT (1932–). Founder of Kripalu Center and originator of Kripalu yoga. Born in Halol, India, he met his guru, Swami Kripalu, at age 15 and came to the U.S. in 1960. He now teaches at Amrit Yoga Institute. Author of *Amrit Yoga & the Yoga Sutras* (2002) and *Amrit Yoga: Explore, Expand and Experience the Spiritual Dimension of Yoga* (2000).

DESIKACHAR, T.K.V. (1938–). Born in Mysore, India, son of T. Krishnamacharya, he began training in yoga with his father while in his 20s. He is the developer of Viniyoga and the author of *Health, Healing and Beyond* (1998) and *The Heart of Yoga: Developing a Personal Practice* (1995).

DOGEN (1200–1253). Japanese Zen master, born in Kyoto, who founded the Soto Zen lineage of Buddhism in Japan. Author of *Shobo-genzo*, a collection of dharma essays.

FARMER, ANGELA. Yoga teacher who was born in England and studied with Iyengar for ten years before developing her own free yoga style using fluid poses for inner exploration. Creator of the video *The Feminine Unfolding* (1999).

FINGER, ALAN (1946–). Born in South Africa, he studied yoga with his father and came to the U.S. in 1976. He is the founder of Yoga Zone in New York City and developer of ISHTA yoga, a style combining Ashtanga, Vinyasa, Iyengar, Kriya and Tantric practices. Author of *The Yoga Zone: Introduction to Yoga* (2000).

FINGER, KAVI YOGIRAJ MANI (1907–). A student of Paramahansa Yogananda, who initiated him into Kriya yoga, and of Swami Sivananda of Rishikesh, he is the father of Alan Finger. He founded the Yoga Teacher's Fellowship in South Africa and spread the teachings of yoga throughout Africa.

GELEK RINPOCHE (1939–   ). Born in Tibet, he was a monk in the largest Tibetan monastery until the Chinese invasion in 1959. Now an American citizen, he is the director of the Jewel Heart Sangha, a Tibetan Buddhist spiritual, cultural, and humanitarian organization. Author of *Good Life, Good Death: Tibetan Wisdom on Reincarnation* (2001).

GOENKA, S.N. (1924–   ). Born and raised in Burma, where he studied with the late Sayagyi U Ba Khin, he has been teaching Vipassana meditation since 1969. He established the Vipassana Research Institute in Igatpuri, India, in 1981 and is the author of *Discourse Summaries: Talks from a Ten-Day Course in Vipassana Meditation* (2000) and *Gracious Flow of Dharma* (1994).

GOLDSTEIN, JOSEPH (1944–   ). Cofounder and resident teacher of the Insight Meditation Society and the Barre Center for Buddhist Studies, in Barre, MA, he studied and practiced intensively in India and Burma. He is the author of many books, including *Insight Meditation: The Practice of Freedom* (1993) and *The Experience of Insight* (1976).

GURUMAYI. *see* **CHIDVILASANANDA.**

HANH, THICH NHAT (1926–   ). Vietnamese Buddhist monk, poet, and peace activist, who came to prominence during the Vietnam War when he urged Buddhist monks and nuns to become active in a movement he called "Socially Engaged Buddhism." He founded Plum Village in France, a Buddhist monastery and Mindfulness practice center for laypeople. His many books include *Vietnam: Lotus in a Sea of Fire* (1967) and *Peace Is Every Step* (1991).

HOLLEMAN, DONA. Student of B.K.S. Iyengar, J. Krishnamurti, and Vanda Scaravelli, she is a yoga teacher who encourages her students to find their own inner teacher. Author of *Dancing the Body of Light* (2000).

IYENGAR, B.K.S. (1918–   ). Originator of Iyengar yoga, he was introduced to yoga at the age of 16 by his sister's husband, T. Krishnamacharya. Iyengar's school, the Ramamani Iyengar Memorial Yoga Institute, was founded in 1974 in Pune, India. He is the author of *Light on Yoga* (1966), *Light on Pranayama* (1981), and other titles.

IYENGAR, GEETA (1944–   ). Daughter of B.K.S. Iyengar and a well-known yoga teacher in her own right, she is trained in Ayurveda and is the author of *Yoga: A Gem for Women* (1990).

JUNG, CARL (1875–1961). Swiss psychiatrist who collaborated with and later broke away from Freud to develop his own school of analytical psychology. His many books include *The Psychology of the Unconscious* (1912) and *Memories, Dreams, Reflections* (1962).

KABIR (15th century). Mystic poet and philosopher born in India around 1398, his work has been popularized in the West by Robert Bly in such books as *Fish in the Sea Is Not Thirsty* (1971).

KLEIN, JEAN (ca. 1916–1998). A prominent Western teacher of advaita, he spent his childhood in Czechoslovakia and the war years in France before embarking on teaching advaita around 1960. He is the author of *Transmission of the Flame* (1990) and *Living Truth* (1995).

KORNFIELD, JACK (1945–   ). Cofounder of Insight Meditation Society and Spirit Rock Meditation Center, he received his Buddhist training in Thailand, Burma, and India and holds a Ph.D. in clinical psychology. Author of *A Path With Heart* (1993) and *After the Ecstasy, the Laundry* (2000).

KRIPALU, SWAMI (1913–1981). Kundalini yoga master, writer, and musician who spent the last four years of his life in the U.S. (1977–1981). Teacher of Yogi Amrit Desai, Swami Kripalu's life and teachings inspired Kripalu yoga. Author of *Science of Meditation* (1977) and *Premyatra: A Pilgrimage of Love* (1981).

KRISHNAMACHARYA, TIRUMALAI (1888–1989). Pioneering Indian yoga master whose work reached the West through his students, B.K.S. Iyengar, Pattabhi Jois, Indra Devi, and T.K.V. Desikachar, who was his son. He worked with the therapeutic applications of yoga and adapted yoga practice to the individual student.

KRISHNAMURTI, J. (1895–1986). Philosopher, spiritual teacher, speaker, and writer, he was born in south India and "discovered" by the Theosophical Society while still a boy. He later disassociated himself from all organized ideologies and religions. Author of many books, including *The Awakening of Intelligence* (1973) and *Think On These Things* (1964).

KRIYANANDA, GOSWAMI. Founder and spiritual head of The Temple of Kriya Yoga in Chicago, he was taught by a devotee of Paramahansa Yogananda. Author of *The Spiritual Science of Kriya Yoga* (1985) and other titles.

LAING, R.D. (1927–1989). British psychiatrist whose unconventional views of mental illness resulted in his coming to public attention in the 1960s. Author of *The Politics of Experience* (1967) and *The Divided Self* (1960).

LEWIS, MURSHID SAMUEL (1896–1971). A spiritual teacher in the Sufi order also ordained as a Zen master, he originated the Dances of Universal Peace. Born in San Francisco, his mentors included Hazrat Inayat Khan. Author of *In the Garden* (1975) and other titles.

MAHARAJI (1957–   ). Sometimes called "the child yogi," he was born Prem Rawal in India. He is the leader of Elan Vital, the successor organization to the Divine Light Mission. He came to the U.S. in 1971 and is the author of *The Living Master* (1978).

MAHARSHI, RAMANA (1879–1950). Indian spiritual teacher and mystic, born in south India. He had an enlightenment experience at age 16, and lived out his life on Arunachala, the hill sacred to Shiva. He was a non-dual teacher of Vedanta, who taught self-inquiry as a path to spiritual awakening. His disciple Ganapathi Muni recorded Ramana's teachings in a work published as the *Sri Ramana Gita* (1954).

MUKTANANDA, SWAMI (1908–1982). Kundalini yoga master and disciple of Swami Nityananda, he came to the West in the 1970s and founded Siddha yoga. He published many books, including the autobiographical *Play of Consciousnes* (1974), and *Where Are You Going?* (1981).

MURSHID. "Spiritual Master, Teacher, Guide, Example;" *see* **LEWIS.**

NYOSHUL KHENPO RINPOCHE (1932–1999). Tibetan Buddhist and Dzogchen master, born in Tibet, fled in 1959. One of the principal teachers of Lama Surya Das, author of *Natural Great Perfection: Dzogchen Teachings and Vajra Songs,* translated by Surya Das (1995).

PATANJALI (second century BCE). Indian sage and compiler of the *Yoga-Sutra*, a collection of 195 aphorisms in which he set out the eight limbs of classical yoga. Few specifics are known about Patanjali's life, but it is thought that the *Yoga-Sutra* was written between 300 and 100 BCE.

PERLS, FREDERICK S. "FRITZ" (1893–1970). Born in Berlin, he was a psychoanalyst best known as the father of Gestalt Therapy. He moved to the U.S. after World War II, organized the Institute of Gestalt Therapy in New York in the 1950s, and worked at Esalen Institute beginning in 1964. He is the author of *Ego, Hunger and Aggression: A Revision of Freud's Theory and Method* (1947) and *Gestalt Therapy Verbatim* (1969).

PUNDIT. *see* **TIGUNAIT.**

RAM DASS (1931–   ). Born Richard Alpert, he was dismissed from teaching at Harvard for his psychedelic research with Timothy Leary. He traveled to India in 1967 where he met his guru, Neem Karoli Baba. He cofounded the Seva Foundation and is the author of the influential book *Be Here Now* (1971) and *Still Here: Embracing Aging, Changing, Dying* (2000).

RAMACHARAKA, YOGI (1862–1932). Probably the pen name of William Walker Atkinson, a lawyer turned yoga teacher who wrote a number of early books on hatha yoga and yoga philosophy including *Inner Teachings of the Philosophies and Religions of India* (1909) and *Advanced Course in Yogic Philosophy* (1904).

ROLF, IDA (1896–1979). Founder of the modality called Structural Integration, later known as Rolfing, a form of body therapy that involves manipulation and repositioning of fascia (connective tissues), and which is said to align and balance the body. Author of *Rolfing: The Integration of Human Structures* (1977).

ROSEN, RICHARD. Senior editor of *International Journal of Yoga Therapy* and deputy director of the Yoga Research and Education Center. He is an Iyengar yoga teacher, contributing editor of *Yoga Journal,* and author of *The Yoga of Breath: A Step-by-Step Guide to Pranayama* (2002).

ROSS, JEAN E. (1916–1996). One of Suzuki Roshi's earliest students in San Francisco, she was the first American women to study at Eiheiji, the oldest monastery of Soto Zen in Japan (1962–63).

RUMI (1207–1273). Sufi poet and mystic, born in what is present-day Afghanistan, he struck up a spiritual friendship with the Sufi devotee Shams of Tabriz. Rumi composed thousands of poems after Shams disappeared. He has been popularized in the West by Coleman Barks in such books as *The Essential Rumi* (1995).

SALZBERG, SHARON. Cofounder of the Insight Meditation Society and the Center for Buddhist Studies, she trained with Buddhist masters in India, Burma, Nepal, Bhutan, and Tibet. Among her titles are *Lovingkindness: The Revolutionary Art of Happiness* (1995) and *Faith: Trusting Your Own Deepest Experience* (2002).

SATCHIDANANDA, SWAMI (1914–2002). Disciple of Swami Sivananda of Rishikesh and others, and founder of Integral Yoga Institutes, he came to the U.S. in 1966 and gained world attention when he gave the invocation at Woodstock in 1969. He founded the Yogaville community in Buckingham, VA, and is the author of *Integral Yoga Hatha* (1970) and other titles.

SCARAVELLI, VANDA. Italian yoga teacher who developed her own unnamed style of yoga that stresses trusting the body's wisdom. She was the teacher of Dona Holleman and of Esther Myers, and author of *Awakening the Spine* (1991).

SEGAL, SUZANNE (1952–1997). California psychologist who had an enlightenment experience in 1982 in which her personal identity disappeared. She was the author of *Collision With the Infinite: A Life Beyond the Personal Self* (1996).

SINGH, CHARAN (1916–1990). Called Maharaj Ji by his followers, Singh was the leader of the Radhasoami Satsang, a school of practical spiritual training founded in India in 1861. Also known as Surat Shabd Yoga, its practice emphasizes attuning to inner, sacred sound.

SIVANANDA, SWAMI (1887–1963). Indian yoga master born Kuppuswami Iyer, he founded the Divine Life Society in Rishikesh in 1936. Although he never went abroad, his teachings were brought to the West by his disciples Swami Satchidananda and Swami Vishnu-Devananda. Author of *Science of Yoga* (18 vols.; 1977) and *Practical Lessons in Yoga* (1978).

STEWART, MARY (1933–   ). Yoga teacher whose style emphasizes the breath, she was a student of Vanda Scaravelli. Her books include *Yoga for Children* (1992) and *Yoga Over 50* (1994).

STUART, MAURINE (1922–1990). Zen teacher and head of Cambridge, (MA) Buddhist Association, she was a disciple of Nakagawa Soen Roshi.

SUMEDHO, AJAHN (1934–   ). Born Robert Jackman in Seattle, WA, he left the U.S. in 1964 and took ordination as a monk in Thailand in 1967. A disciple of Achaan Chah, he is now abbot of Amaravati Buddhist Centre near London and author of *The Mind and the Way: Buddhist Reflections on Life* (1995).

SUNG ZHAN (also spelled **SEUNG SAHN**). One of the first Korean Zen masters to live and teach in the U.S. He came to the U.S. in 1972, eventually founding Zen centers in Providence, RI, and other U.S. cities. Author of *Dropping Ashes on the Buddha* (1976) and *Only Don't Know* (1982).

SUWAT, AJAAN. Thai forest meditation teacher who helped bring the Thai forest traditions to the U.S. Author of *A Fistful of Sand* (1999).

SUZUKI, SHUNRYU, ROSHI (1904–1971). Japanese Zen priest of the Soto lineage. Founder and first abbot of the San Francisco Zen Center and author of *Zen Mind, Beginner's Mind* (1970).

SWAMI. *see* **AJAYA, AMBIKANANDA SARASWATI, CHETANANDA, CHIDAN-ANDA, KRIPALU, MUKTANANDA, SIVANANDA, VISHNU-DEVANANDA.**

TAGORE, RABINDRANATH (1861–1941). Indian poet, writer, and philosopher who won the Nobel Prize for Literature in 1913. Considered one of modern India's great writers, he published over 50 volumes of poetry, along with short stories and novels, including *Gitanjali* (1910) and *The Post Office* (1912).

THAKAR, VIMALA (ca.1922–   ). Indian spiritual master and meditation teacher strongly influenced by Krishnamurti and Gandhi. From the 1960s to the '80s, she taught meditation in over 35 countries. Her books include *On an Eternal Voyage* (1972), about her experiences with Krishnamurti, and *Blossoms of Friendship* (1975).

THIRD ANCESTOR OF ZEN (sixth century). Seng-T'san, or Sosan, a wandering monk in China whose poem *Hsin Shin Ming* is one of Zen's earliest writings. He is also known for the statement "The Great Way is not difficult for those who have no preferences."

TIGUNAIT, PUNDIT RAJMANI (1953–   ). Spiritual head of the Himalayan Institute in Honesdale, PA, and successor of Swami Rama, he is the author of many books, including *Himalayan Masters: A Living Tradition* (2002) and *At the Eleventh Hour: The Biography of Swami Rama* (2001).

TRUNGPA, CHOGYAM, RINPOCHE (1939–1987). Meditation master and teacher of the Kagyu lineage, he pioneered Tibetan Buddhist teaching in the West. Born in Tibet, he fled during the Chinese invasion of 1959, studied in England, and came to the U.S. in 1970. Founder of Naropa Institute, he is the author of *Cutting Through Spiritual Materialism* (1973) and many other works.

VISHNU-DEVANANDA, SWAMI (1929–1993). Disciple of Swami Sivananda of Rishikesh, he traveled to the West and founded the International Sivananda Yoga Vedanta Centers, headquartered in Quebec. Author of *The Complete Illustrated Book of Yoga* (1959).

YOGANANDA, PARAMAHANSA (1893–1952). Born Mukunda Lal Ghosh, he was a disciple of Sri Yukteswar Giri, who encouraged him to take the message of yoga to the West. He arrived in the U.S. in 1920 and founded Self-Realization Fellowship in 1935. Author of *Autobiography of a Yogi* (1946).

YOGI. *see* **BHAJAN, DESAI, RAMACHARAKA.**

ZAHN. *see* **SUNG ZAHN.**

ZIMMER, HEINRICH (1890–1943). German-born scholar, specializing in the philosophy and myth of India, his works were edited by Joseph Campbell. He is the author of *The Philosophies of India* (1951) and *Myths and Symbols in Indian Art and Civilization* (1946).

Grateful acknowledgment is made to the following sources of information for the terms and teachers in the glossary, along with many individual and organizational Web sites:

Encyclopedia of Eastern Philosophy and Religion: Buddhism, Hinduism, Taoism, Zen. Boston: Shambhala, 1994.

Feuerstein, Georg. *The Shambhala Encyclopedia of Yoga.* Boston: Shambhala, 1997.

———. *The Yoga Tradition: Its History, Literature, Philosophy, and Practice.* Prescott, Ariz.: Hohm Press, 1998.

Hinnells, John R., editor. *Who's Who of World Religions.* New York: Simon & Schuster, 1992.

Melton, J. Gordon. *Religious Leaders of America.* 2d ed. Detroit: Gale Group, 1999.

Rengarajan, T. *Dictionary of Hinduism.* New Delhi: Oxford & IBH Publishing, 1999.

Sarley, Dinabandhu and Ila. *The Essentials of Yoga.* New York: Dell, 1999.

Seekers Glossary of Buddhism. New York: Sutra Translation Committee, 1998.

Contributors' Publications, Recordings, and Web sites

RAMA BERCH

Yoga in Every Moment (Master Yoga Foundation)
Svaroopa Yoga: The Primary Practice (VHS)
Yoga for Your Back (VHS)
www.masteryoga.org

SYLVIA BOORSTEIN

Pay Attention, for Goodness' Sake: Practicing the Perfections of the Heart: the Buddhist Path of Kindness (Ballantine, 2002)
The Courage to Be Happy: Jewish/Buddhist Teaching Stories on Gratitude, Compassion, and Mindful Awakening (audio) (Sounds True, 2000)
Road Sage: Mindfulness Techniques for Drivers (audio) (Sounds True, 1999)
That's Funny, You Don't Look Buddhist: On Being a Faithful Jew and a Passionate Buddhist (Harper SanFrancisco, 1998)
It's Easier Than You Think: The Buddhist Way to Happiness (HarperSanFrancisco, 1997)
Don't Just Do Something, Sit There: A Mindfulness Retreat with Sylvia Boorstein (HarperSanFrancisco, 1996)
www.spiritrock.org

MAYA BREUER

www.mayabreuer.com

EDWARD ESPE BROWN

Not Always So, Practicing the True Spirit of Zen by Shunryu Suzuki, edited by Edward Espe Brown (HarperCollins, 2002)
The Greens Cookbook with Deborah Madison (Broadway Books, 2001)
The Tassajara Recipe Book with Alice Waters (Random House, 2000)
La Cocina Zen (Integral Publishing, 2000)
Tomato Blessings and Radish Teachings: Finding Your Way in the Kitchen: Stories and Recipes (Riverhead, 1997)
The Organic Gourmet: Recipes and Resources from a Seasonal Kitchen with Barbara Kahn (Frog Ltd., 1995)
The Tassajara Bread Book (Shambhala, 1995)
Tassajara Cooking: (Random House, 1986)
www.yogazen.com

STEPHEN COPE

Yoga and the Quest for the True Self (Bantam, 2000)
Yoga for Emotional Flow (audio) (Sounds True, 2003)
Kripalu Dynamic Yoga (VHS)
www.kripalu.org

ANNE CUSHMAN

From Here to Nirvana: The Yoga Journal Guide to Spiritual India with Jerry Jones (Riverhead, 1999)

LAMA SURYA DAS

Letting Go of the Person You Used to Be: Lessons on Loss, Change, and Spiritual Transformation (Broadway, 2003)

Awakening the Buddhist Heart: Integrating Love, Meaning, and Connection into Every Part of Your Life (Broadway, 2001)

Awakening to the Sacred: Creating a Spiritual Life from Scratch (Broadway, 2000)

Tibetan Dream Yoga (audio) (Sounds True, 2000)

Natural Meditation (video) (Sounds True, 2002)

Buddhism in America (audio) with Allione Tsultrim and Stephen Batchelor (Sounds True, 2000)

Schlepping Towards Enlightenment (audio) (Hay House, 1999)

Awakening the Buddha Within: Tibetan Wisdom for the Western World (Broadway, 1998)

Natural Perfection: Teachings, Meditations, and Chants in the Dzogchen Tradition of Tibet (audio) with Nyoshul Khenpo (Snow Lion Publications, 1995)

www.dzogchen.org

DONNA FARHI

Bringing Yoga to Life: The Everyday Practice of Enlightened Living (HarperSanFrancisco, 2003)

The Breathing Book: Good Health and Vitality Through Essential Breath Work (Henry Holt, 1996)

Yoga Mind, Body & Spirit: A Return to Wholeness (Henry Holt, 2000)

www.donnafarhi.co.nz

RICHARD FAULDS

Kripalu Yoga: A Guide to Practice On & Off the Mat (Bantam, 2004)

www.kripalu.org

LILIAS FOLAN

Lilias Yoga Complete (audio) (Audio Renaissance, 1994)

Lilias: Yoga for Experienced Students (audio) (St. Martin's, 1988)

Lilias, Yoga and Your Life (Macmillan, 1981)

Lilias, Yoga and You (Bantam, 1983)

Inner Smile (audio) (Relaxation Company, 1998)

Rest, Relax and Sleep (audio) (Rudra, 1992)

Lilias' Flowing Postures (VHS)

Lilias' Yoga Workout Series (VHS)

Lilias' Evening Workout for Beginners (VHS)

Lilias' Target Toning for Beginners (VHS)

Lilias' Alive with Yoga (VHS)

Lilias' Discover Gentle Moments (VHS)

www.liliasyoga.com

JOHN FRIEND

Yoga Alignment and Form (VHS)

Yoga for Meditators (VHS)

Anusara 101 (audio)

Anusara Yoga: Teacher Training Manual

Anusara Yoga Essentials (audio)

www.anusara.com

ROBERT HALL

Out of Nowhere (Running Wolf Press, 2000)

www.eldharma.com

JUDITH HANSON LASATER

Relax and Renew: Restful Yoga for Stressful Times (Rodmell Press, 1995)

Living Your Yoga: Finding the Spiritual in Everyday Life (Rodmell Press, 2000)

www.judithlasater.com

CYNDI LEE

Yoga Body, Buddha Mind (Riverhead, 2004

Om Yoga: A Guide to Daily Practice (Chronicle, 2002)

Om: Yoga in a Box for Couples: Beginner Level (audio) (Hay House, 2002)

Om Yoga in a Box: Intermediate Level (audio) (Hay House, 2002)

Om Yoga in a Box: Basic Level (audio) (Hay House, 2002)

Om Yoga Flash Cards (Hay House, 2002)

OM at Home: A Yoga Journal (Chronicle, 2003)

www.omyoga.com

RICHARD MILLER

www.nondual.com

PHILLIP MOFFITT

www.lifebalance.org

ESTHER MYERS

Yoga and You: Energizing and Relaxing Yoga for New and Experienced Teachers (Shambhala, 1997; Random House Canada)

Hands-On Manual for Teachers (self-pub.)

www.estheryoga.com

LARRY ROSENBERG

Breath by Breath: The Liberating Practice of Insight Meditation (Shambhala, 1999)

Living in the Light of Death: On the Art of Being Truly Alive with David Guy (Shambhala, 2001)

www.cimc.info

MU SOENG

The Diamond Sutra: Transforming the Way We Perceive the World (Wisdom Pub., 2000)

PATRICIA SULLIVAN

Shtira and Sukham in Sirsasana and Sarvangasana: A Step by Step Practice and Teaching Manual (self-pub., 2003)

ROD STRYKER

Yoga for Longevity (VHS)

3 Meditations to Live By (CD)

www.pureyoga.com

PATRICIA WALDEN

The Woman's Book of Yoga and Health: A Lifelong Guide to Wellness with Linda Sparrowe (Shambhala, 2003)

Yoga Basics with Patricia Walden (DVD)

Yoga Journal's Practice Series (VHS)

a.m./p.m. Yoga for Beginners Video Set (VHS)

www.yogawisdom.com

LARRY YANG

Contributor to *Friends on the Path* by Thich Nhat Hanh (Parallax Press, 2002)

Acknowledgments

It has been said — that "the next generation of gurus in America will be communities." What this means, I think, is that in the future, the wisdom of the contemplative traditions will inhere not in any one charismatic individual, but in the community as a whole. In these new communities, the work of transformation will be fully collaborative. This book is in so many ways a manifestation of that very vision. Its production has been collaborative in every way, and whatever wisdom is in it has been group wisdom. The many small and large miracles of generosity that have arisen throughout the course of its development have demonstrated to me the ways in which a new, nonsectarian community of teachers and practitioners already exists in America. I am inspired by and grateful for this spirit of collaboration, and for the contributions of so many.

First I would like to thank the twenty-four American teachers who generously gave of their time to contribute essays and interviews to this volume. All of the work published here is fresh, and is performed out of love for the inquiry and without any compensation. Each contributor has wrestled deeply and honorably with the complex questions that I posed. As a result, these pieces have the kind of vitality that makes a difference in readers' lives, and I believe that together they will make a difference in how we think about contemplative practice. Thank you, my dear friends and colleagues!

The team at Storey Publishing has proved that enlightenment is not exclusive to the halls of contemplative practice. It is alive and well in publishing. Particularly, I would like to thank Deborah Balmuth, editorial director at Storey, whose vision, energy, courage and vast competence have made this volume possible — along with the support and genius of Publisher Janet Harris, President Pam Art, Art Director Cindy McFarland, Designer Susi Oberhelman, Book Builder Jen Jepson Smith, Photo Manager Laurie Figary, Tape Transcriber Chris Meyer, and Publicist Dianne Cutillo.

Though my name appears on the front of this book as Editor, the full truth is that the editing of this volume has been a collaborative — and exhilarating — experience from start to finish. I wish particularly to thank the incredibly skillful Atma Jo Ann Levitt, Bhavani Lorraine Nelson, and Rachel Barenblat for their tireless contributions over the course of many months. In addition, may I praise the excellent work of Danna Faulds, who brought all her formidable skills to bear on the glossary and list of Key Teachers — probably in themselves worth the price of the book — as well as the index.

The Kripalu Center for Yoga & Health, and the Kripalu Community at large, has supported this endeavor from the start. In particular let me thank Sudhir Jonathan Foust, president of Kripalu Yoga Fellowship, and Shobhan Richard Faulds, chairman of the Board of Kripalu Yoga Fellowship, for their visionary leadership in helping to launch the new Kripalu Books Imprint, of which this volume is the first manifestation. In addition, Al Meyerer, Vice

President of Programming; Cathy Husid, Director of Publicity; Andrea Mather, Editor of the Kripalu Program Guide; Jayme Hummer, Editorial Assistant; Derek Hansen, Design Coordinator; and Aruni Nan Futoronsky, Director of Retreat and Renewal have each contributed gifts essential to the completion of this project. Adam Mastoon made the beautiful photograph for the cover and consulted on other photographic issues with his usual expertise and visual intelligence.

And finally, on behalf of the entire creative team, I wish to dedicate the merits of this book to the happiness of all beings.

Photo Credits

Sylvia Boorstein (p. 12) by Christine Alicino; Larry Yang (p. 28) © Thomas Heinser; Patricia Walden (p. 82) © Jonathan Pozniak; Konda Mason (p. 108) by Cat Jiminez; Cyndi Lee (p. 128) © Constance Wallace; Richard Miller (p. 136) by Jennie Miller; Maya Breuer (p. 162) by Rhoda Kitzner Bailey; Richard Faulds (p. 180) by Mary Schjeldahl; Lilias Folan (p. 192) by Circe Hamilton; Judith Hanson Lasater (p.212) by Seth Affoumado; Rod Stryker (p. 240) by Bud Symes; Robert Hall (p. 256) by José Alvaro Colindres; Patricia Sullivan (p. 270) by Ed Brown; Stephen Cope (p. 284) by Adam Mastoon.

Index

Note: page numbers in **bold** print denote photographs

Vedanta, 54, 194, 230, 304
Vedas, 252, 304
Viniyoga, 100, 145, 304
vinyasa, 135, 304
Vipassana
    and sensations, 264, 267
    definition of, 176, 304
    experience of, 43, 264
    Krishnamurti's teaching, 57
    practiced with yoga, 175
    retreats with S.N. Goenka, 77
    teachers in America, 3, 100, 258
Vishnu Devananda, Swami, 194, 225, 314
Visuddhimagga, 6, 304

Walden, Patrica, **82**–97, 318
Wicca, 222, 304
witness consciousness, 200, 203
Wu-men-kwan, 209, 304

Yang, Larry, **28**–37, 318
yoga
    alignment in, 68
    and aging, 202, 279
    and Buddhism, 44, 58, 175
    and depression, 85–86, 202
    and mastectomy, 66, 70–71
    and work, 276–277
    definition of, 304–305
    for women, 84
    goal of, 49, 67, 139–140, 216, 254
    Krishnamurti's practice of, 57
    no guarantees in, 67
    number of practitioners, 3
    perfection in, 6, 49–50, 139
    purpose of, 186
    self-observation in, 118, 187–188, 200,
        203
    TV shows, 194–196
    See also asana; meditation; practice
yoga, effects of practicing,
    appreciation of life, 51, 189, 219, 250
    attuning to sensations, 43, 48, 142,
        144, 148

awakening witness, 200, 203
awareness of body, 47–51, 135, 187
change in brain chemistry, 86–87
compassion, 113, 218
effortless being, 190–191, 293
embracing imperfection, 50
emotional release, 134
everything OK, 292
exhilaration, 245
fear, decrease in, 140, 153–154, 250
freedom, increase of, 254
healing separation, 113
heart opening, 45–46, 81, 219
joy, 45, 142, 250
present to what is, 190, 279, 291
purification, 187–188
relaxing into life, 133, 190
safety, creation of, 88, 155, 188
self-awareness, 187–188
self-soothing, 89, 132
tension release, 274
yoga nidra, 142, 305
Yoga-Sutra of Patanjali, 6–7, 238, 244, 305
Yoga Tantric Institute, 242
Yoga, Youth & Reincarnation (Stearn), 225,
    273–274, 305
Yogananda, Paramahansa, 167, 225, 242,
    248, 281, 314
Yogatopia, 242
yogin, 6, 305

Zen
    and daily life, 102–103
    and teachers, 283
    attraction to, 101
    definition of, 305
    effects of practicing, 125–126, 207–208
    in China, 117–118
    "not knowing" in, 208
    "practical–minded," 117
    seated meditation in, 121, 207
Zen Center of Los Angeles, 40, 43
Zimmer, Heinrich, *Philosophies of India,* 11,
    315